AF743993

APPROACHES TO HYSTERECTOMY

Edited by **Zouhair O. Amarin**

Approaches to Hysterectomy
http://dx.doi.org/10.5772/59454
Edited by Zouhair O. Amarin

Contributors

Chrisostomos Sofoudis, Zhiqing Liang, Ambrogio P Londero, Serena Bertozzi, Ralph J Lellé, Angelo Calcagno, Arrigo Fruscalzo, Luca Martella, Giulio Bertola, Giorgio Giorda, Georgios Androutsopoulos, Georgios Decavalas, Georgios Michail, Dimitris Karnabatidis, Eugenio Volpi, Giulia Moggio, Daniel Dimitrios Paramythiotis, Kimberly Kim, Christopher Balogun-Lynch, Tahira Aziz Javaid, Zouhair Amarin

Published by InTech

Janeza Trdine 9, 51000 Rijeka, Croatia

© The Editor(s) and the Author(s) 2015

The moral rights of the editor(s) and the author(s) have been asserted.
All rights to the book as a whole are reserved by InTech. The book as a whole (compilation) cannot be reproduced, distributed or used for commercial or non-commercial purposes without InTech's written permission. Enquiries concerning the use of the book should be directed to InTech's rights and permissions department (permissions@intechopen.com).
Violations are liable to prosecution under the governing Copyright Law.

Individual chapters of this publication are distributed under the terms of the Creative Commons Attribution 3.0 Unported License which permits commercial use, distribution and reproduction of the individual chapters, provided the original author(s) and source publication are appropriately acknowledged. More details and guidelines concerning content reuse and adaptation can be found at http://www.intechopen.com/copyright-policy.html.

Notice

Statements and opinions expressed in the chapters are these of the individual contributors and not necessarily those of the editors or publisher. No responsibility is accepted for the accuracy of information contained in the published chapters. The publisher assumes no responsibility for any damage or injury to persons or property arising out of the use of any materials, instructions, methods or ideas contained in the book.

Publishing Process Manager Iva Lipovic

Technical Editor InTech DTP team

Cover InTech Design team

First published November, 2015

Printed in Croatia

Additional hard copies can be obtained from orders@intechopen.com

Approaches to Hysterectomy, Edited by Zouhair O. Amarin

p. cm.

ISBN 978-953-51-2199-2

We are IntechOpen, the world's leading publisher of Open Access books

Built by scientists, for scientists

3,800+
Open access books available

116,000+
International authors and editors

120M+
Downloads

151
Countries delivered to

Our authors are among the
Top 1%
most cited scientists

12.2%
Contributors from top 500 universities

WEB OF SCIENCE™

Selection of our books indexed in the Book Citation Index
in Web of Science™ Core Collection (BKCI)

Interested in publishing with us?
Contact book.department@intechopen.com

Numbers displayed above are based on latest data collected.
For more information visit www.intechopen.com

For EU product safety concerns:
IN TECH d.o.o., Prolaz Marije Krucifikse Kozulić 3, 51000 Rijeka, Croatia, info@intechopen.com or visit our website at intechopen.com.

Meet the editor

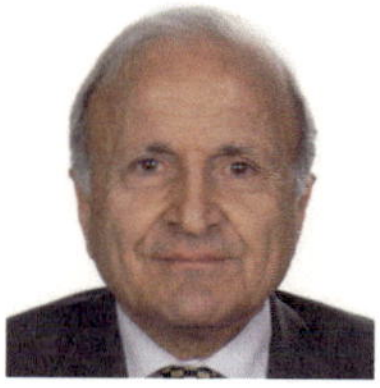

Zouhair O. Amarin is a Professor of Obstetrics and Gynaecology at the Jordan University of Science and Technology. He was a Lecturer at the University of Glasgow, Senior Lecturer at the University of Nottingham, and Dean of the Faculty of Medicine at Mutah University. Professor Amarin is a Fellow of the Royal College of Obstetricians and Gynaecologists and the Faculty of Public Health, London. He holds a master's degree in medical science, Glasgow, and in medical education, Maastricht. He is a pioneer of in vitro fertilization (IVF), and he was the first to develop microsurgical epididymis sperm aspiration for clinical use. He discovered a surgical procedure for critical ovarian hyperstimulation syndrome. Professor Amarin has published more than 100 papers and has received eight awards.

Contents

Preface

Excellence in the dynamic art of surgery always commands admiration and respect. The enthusiasm of this should be shared. In so doing, the secrets of perfection, which depend not only on scientific knowledge but also on manual dexterity, are revealed.

As with any surgery, a hysterectomy is both patient- and procedure-specific. Today, there are a number of advanced options that feature shorter hospital stays, less postoperative pain and a quick return to normal activity.

The long-standing techniques of hysterectomy are well described in many textbooks, but chapters on alternatives to hysterectomy and laparoscopic surgery in this book deal with relatively new techniques. Nevertheless, these latter topics can involve fine judgement for their appropriate use in a problem-oriented approach.

Even when the correct operation has been adequately performed, there is always the risk that complications will arise. The last chapter on peripartum hysterectomy includes some technical details acquired from experience that cover such problems where the recognition of their incipient signs can initiate the correct action. In an emergency, the best management has to be a combination of action and adequate knowledge and skills.

I would like to thank all the authors for their invaluable efforts and contributions. Thanks also go to Ana Pantar, Ivona Lovrić and Iva Lipović, Publishing Process Managers, for their support and advice.

Professor Zouhair O. Amarin
Department of Obstetrics and Gynaecology
Jordan University of Science and Technology
Jordan

Section 1

Comparative Analyses of Symptoms in Women Before and After Hysterectomy

Chapter 1

Comparative Analyses of Pain, Depressed Mood and Sleep Disturbance Symptoms in Women before and after Hysterectomy

Kimberly H. Kim

Additional information is available at the end of the chapter

Abstract

Hysterectomy affects several aspects of a woman's health, and persons considering a surgery should be aware of its effectiveness for relief of symptoms and long term effects on quality of life. The aims of the study were to examine pain, depressed mood, and sleep disturbance symptoms of women before and six weeks after hysterectomy; compare the physiological and social variables related to the symptoms, and examine the levels of symptom severity between abdominal vs vaginal hysterectomy. A pre and post measures study collected data from a prospective sample of 26 of the 36 culturally diverse women who were scheduled for hysterectomy using subjective questionnaires and objective wrist actigraphy monitoring for sleep and wake time. Results indicated that the majority of participants reported moderate amounts of pain before surgery however an average pain score did not vary over time. Depressed mood scores in women with laparoscopic vaginal hysterectomy significantly decreased from the baseline to six weeks after surgery, showing less severity of depression after surgery. Compared to the baseline measures, wrist actigraphy recordings showed increases in the numbers of awakening, wake after sleep onset and day time sleep during six weeks after surgery indicating that women had more sleep disturbance postoperatively. However, compared to women who had the abdominal surgery, those with vaginal hysterectomy reported a significantly severe sleep disturbance at six weeks after surgery; and younger women experienced more wake time at night. Evidence based findings indicated that hysterectomy relieved pain however women continued to experience disturbed sleep patterns six weeks after surgery, suggesting further research is needed in light of women's health.

Keywords: Hysterectomy, pain, depressed mood, sleep disturbance, TAH and LAVH

INTECH
open science | open minds

© 2015 The Author(s). Licensee InTech. This chapter is distributed under the terms of the Creative Commons Attribution License (http://creativecommons.org/licenses/by/3.0), which permits unrestricted use, distribution, and reproduction in any medium, provided the original work is properly cited.

1. Introduction

Hysterectomy relieves preoperative symptoms including heavy bleeding and pain; however it may carry a substantial risk of morbidity such as sleep disturbance and depressed mood. Current evidences indicate that after a hysterectomy, women experience further complications during the recovery period that might vary with the type of surgical procedure. During this period, the quantity and quality of sleep as well as other symptoms such as pain, anxiety, and depressive symptoms might be influenced by various demographic and biopsychosocial factors. Despite limited evidence that sleep problems may occur frequently during the recovery period, only a few researchers have systematically examined symptom outcomes in women after hysterectomy. This study investigated the pain, depressed mood, and sleep disturbance symptoms experienced by women before and after hysterectomy and compared their multi-dimensional biopsychosocial variables including surgical procedures related to the symptoms.

2. Literature review

Hysterectomy was one of the most common gynecological surgeries in the United States [1-4]. According to the National Center of Health Statistics, approximately 600,000 hysterectomies were performed annually in the United States. It also was one of the most frequently performed surgeries among women all over the world with annual rates of 50,000 in Canada [5-6], 1.8/1000 in Denmark [1], 4.1/1000 in Finland [1], and 11,000 in Portugal [4]. The most common indications for a hysterectomy comprised of leiomyoma, endometriosis, prolapse of the uterus, cancer of the reproductive tract, adenomyosis, fibroids, and heavy bleeding [7-9]. Varying rates of surgical cases were reported in literature, however approximately 40% of hysterectomies were elective [10], and 90% were operated for a benign condition [11].

A hysterectomy could be done in various ways; such as vaginal hysterectomy, abdominal hysterectomy, laparoscopic assisted vaginal or total hysterectomy, and robotic assisted hysterectomy. The choice might depend on diagnoses and physicians' ability to perform procedures on their patients. Total abdominal hysterectomy (TAH) was performed more commonly for myomas [12] and presence of malignancy [13] however it was associated with a worse patient experience relative to the other types of procedures [14]. In a study, 60% underwent TAH, and those women experienced higher levels of pain and depressed mood after TAH compared to laparoscopic assisted vaginal hysterectomy [15]. Li and colleagues [16] claimed that both procedures had similar efficacy and morbidity rates for women with cervical cancer. Susini and colleagues [17] argued that laparoscopic assisted vaginal hysterectomy (LAVH) had both advantages and disadvantages. An advantage of LAVH was the ability to inspect the tissue with laparoscopy once vaginal cuff closure was completed; however the complication rate did not exceed that of TAH when performed by well-trained physicians. Robotic assisted surgery for endometrial cancer has further been shown to reduce blood loss, while maintaining the benefits of laparoscopic techniques [18-19] however its lengthy preparation and operating time would contribute to an exorbitant price and cause cost inefficiency.

Although the research addressed the substantial numbers of positive effects such as relief of physical symptoms and improvements of social and psychological functioning, the appropriateness of using hysterectomy to treat non-malignant conditions remained controversial [10]. Research showed the possible reasons of negative physical and psychological outcomes after hysterectomy; such as depression [20-21], sleep disturbance and fatigue [22, 7], pelvic pain [23], sexual dysfunction [24-25, 11], and urinary incontinence or symptoms [26].

Sleep disturbance is one of the most prevalent symptoms following hysterectomy. Kim and Lee [7] reported that three weeks after surgery, women's self-reported sleep disturbance was significantly higher than baseline. Similarly, after adjustment for factors such as current psychological, vasomotor, and somatic symptoms and waking frequently at night to use the toilet, a study on self-reported sleep difficulty during the menopausal transition demonstrated that women with hysterectomy remained at higher risk for moderate sleep difficulty [27]. Another study evaluated the sleep patterns before gynecologic surgery that indicated sleep quality was only impaired in the very last night before surgery [28]. Moreover, no significant association between the nature of the planned surgery and preoperative sleep characteristics was shown in the study. A study by researchers [29] compared two groups receiving treatments, one receiving the GnRH agonist and other receiving hysterectomy for treatment of dysfunctional uterine bleeding in premenopausal women and concluded that there was no significant differences existed between two treatment groups in sleep disorders after two-years of follow up.

Pain before and after hysterectomy has been discussed in the literature. Although Solnik and Munro [30] suggested that women experiencing chronic pelvic pain should be counseled against hysterectomy until a more clear etiology was identified, Tiwana and colleague [31] claimed that women with chronic pelvic pain must consider hysterectomy. It is quite common for women to experience chronic pain following hysterectomy. Brandsborg and colleagues [1] argued that chronic pain was prevalent in women with hysterectomy; on their study, 5-32% of women reported to experience pain. Chronic pelvic pain persisted after surgery in 22% of cases [32] and 19% of cases that needed a further intervention to cure this problem [12]. Furthermore, Darnall and Li [33] reported that 29% of the female sample (n = 323) aged between18 and 45 at a chronic pain clinic reported to experience pain: They suggested that hysterectomy might confer risk for pain-related dysfunction and opioid prescription in women 45 years of age and younger. Hysterectomy also was used to treat chronic pelvic pain in the past. In a comparative study of pre-hysterectomy cases, pelvic pain and abdominal pain were reduced five years post hysterectomy [34]. However, several studies demonstrated that in the absence of any obvious pathology, 21-40% of women undergoing hysterectomy to treat chronic pelvic pain might continue to experience pain after the surgery [23], no more than 60-70% might achieve significant pain relief, and 3-5% might suffer worsening of pain or had new onsets of pain [35]. Therefore, it was suggested that women with chronic pelvic pain could consider hysterectomy [31] if they had pelvic varices and were ruled out having non-reproductive causes of pain after a careful pre-operative assessment [23,35].

In regards to pain after hysterectomy, researchers examined whether the severity of acute postoperative pain differed between laparoscopic (LH) or laparoscopically assisted vaginal hysterectomy (LAVH) and vaginal hysterectomy, and found LH was associated with reduced need of analgesics and lower acute pain scores than LAVH [36]. A study in Finland comparing hysterectomy with levonorgestrel-releasing intrauterine system (LNG-IUS) as a treatment for menorrhagia showed that both treatments reduced lower abdominal pain: However, only LNG-IUS use, not hysterectomy, had beneficial effects on back pain [37]. In a study on predictors of acute postsurgical pain in women undergoing hysterectomy due to benign disorders, Pinto and colleagues [4] found that younger age, pre-surgical pain, pain due to other causes, and pain catastrophizing appeared to be the main predictors of pain severity at 48 hours after the operation, while presurgical anxiety also predicted pain intensity after surgery. Their findings revealed the joint influence of demographic, clinical, and psychological factors on postsurgical pain intensity and severity.

In addition to the physical outcomes, much has been written about the possible psychological effects from hysterectomy. 50% of women had obvious abnormal emotions before hysterectomy, and the surgery could cause strong mental stress reactions [21]. Of the statistics, however, women with hysterectomy were not higher in negative affect or negative attitudes toward aging and menopause compared to those without hysterectomy [38]. In a study on 113 women during an eight-week post hysterectomy period, Cohen and colleagues [2] found the significant overall positive changes in anxiety, depression, and hostility: They indicated that the positive changes could be due to women's high self-esteem, which might partially be attributed to the high educational level of the sample. The findings from the study by Farquhar et al. [34] also showed lower depression scores five years following hysterectomy. Nonetheless, Sehlo and Ramadani [20] found that the prevalence of major depressive episode (MDE) was significantly higher in women having hysterectomy compared with women having cholecystectomy. Moreover, the prevalence and severity of MDE was significantly higher in the nullipara group than the multipara group. They declared that hysterectomy increased the risk of MDE that should be diagnosed and treated promptly [20]. Ewalds-Kvist and associates [39] also found that married nullipara suffered from enhanced depression post-surgery.

When evaluating the relationship between hysterectomy and the psychological health afterwards, Cooper, Mishra, Hardy, & Kuh [40] emphasized the importance to take previous psychological status into account: Their findings suggested that women who underwent hysterectomy at a young age might require more support than those who maintained good psychological health in middle age. Similarly, Vandyk, Brenner, Tranmer, and Kerkhof [41] also found that young women with high levels of anxiety and pain that needed a hysterectomy were at high risk of experiencing psychological distress before and after their operation.

The association between hysterectomy and psychological outcomes has aroused the interest of the researcher not only in the United States but outside the US. Researchers in Japan demonstrated that depressed women had a higher incidence of hysterectomy and/or oophorectomy than non-depressed women [42]. By comparing mastectomy patients with hysterectomy patients in a study conducted in Turkey, Keskin & Gumus [25] found that mastectomy patients were more depressive while hysterectomy patients demonstrated more problems in expression of emotions as well as greater sexual problems and difficulties with spousal relationships. Wang, Lambert, & Lambert [43] demonstrated a study on 105 Chinese women with hysterectomy before their scheduled discharge: The findings showed that 4.8% experienced depression; and the best predictors of depression were self-blame and employment status. These results imply that besides physical and psychological factors, social and economic well-being of the post-hysterectomy women were affected.

Without complications, most women with a LAVH require a few weeks of recovery time, however those who undergo an abdominal hysterectomy may require six to eight weeks of longer recovery periods. This study aimed to examine symptoms experienced by women with hysterectomy; compared their perceived pain, depressed mood and sleep disturbance symptoms before and six weeks after hysterectomy; and examined the relationships between their symptoms and biopsychosocial variables including types of surgical procedures, TAH vs LAVH.

3. Methods

The pre and post measures study examined pain, depressed mood and sleep disturbance symptoms experienced by a sample of 26 culturally diverse women before and after hysterectomy and evaluated the relationship between their symptoms and biopsychosocial contextual variables. After describing the women's experience of pain, depressed mood and disturbed sleep, the symptoms were compared to determine the differences in symptom severity between two surgical procedures; total abdominal vs. laparoscopic hysterectomy.

3.1. Research participants and procedures

The Institutional Review Board on Human Research approved the study. The inclusion criteria included: (a) women above 30 years of age, (b) no history of pregnancy or surgery for the past one year, (c) no history of mental illnesses, and (d) no history taking psychotropic drugs in the past one year. Potential participants were accessed through the flyer provided by the investigator in the two women's clinics at two to three weeks prior to surgery. Once women expressed an interest in participating in the study, they were asked to call the investigator who would provide the details of the study and obtain informed consent, their health history, and baseline data that included physiologic, psychological and social variables as well as sleep-wake patterns and symptoms. They were given information about instructions on how to manage a wrist actigraph although this instruction was repeated at the time of wearing the actigraph by the researcher as participants needed to wear a wrist actigraph for 48 hours, between three days to two weeks before their scheduled surgery. Once discharged from the hospital, women were asked to wear the wrist actigraph in their home to monitor activity continuously for 48 hours at six weeks after surgery. At each time point, they were also asked to complete standardized questionnaires that measure pain and depressed mood. Participants were informed to record their sleep and wake times on a diary. Standardized questionnaires used for this study took approximately 15 minutes to complete. After each 48-hour session, the investigator collected the wrist actigraph and diary from the participant's home.

3.2. Measurements

The women's biopsychosocial and symptom variables were evaluated using standardized questionnaires completed by participants and objective actigraphy data for sleep efficiency and sleep-wake patterns. Physiologic factors included age at preoperative baseline as well as whether the surgery was a laparotomy approach to total abdominal hysterectomy (TAH) or laparoscopic assisted vaginal hysterectomy/vaginal hysterectomy (LAVH). Social factors included ethnicity (African/Black, Asian, Caucasian/European, or Hispanic), marital status (single, married, divorced, or widowed), education (graduates of high school, college, or post-graduate work), employment (full- or part-time, homemaker, or retired), and numbers of children. These data were collected as part of the health history baseline data.

Symptom measures included pain, depressed mood and sleep disturbance. Pain was measured at baseline and six weeks after surgery with the Wisconsin Brief Pain Inventory (BPI) to address multidimensional aspects of pain. Participants were asked to circle a number to describe the extent to which pain interfered with various activities from 0 (does not interfere) to 10 (completely interfere), during the past week. Internal consistency reliability of the severity and interference subscales on the BPI revealed Cronbach alpha coefficients of 0.89 and 0.90 in this sample.

Depressed mood was measured with the 21-item Beck Depression Inventory (BDI) pre-operatively and at six weeks after surgery by having the participant rate their perception of mood intensity from 0 (absence of depression) to 3 (the most severe depression). The BDI has established test-retest reliability ranges of 0.74 to 0.95 with elderly and depressive subjects. Internal consistency (Cronbach alpha coefficient) for this study was 0.93 preoperatively. The cutoffs scores were 0–13 (minimal depression); 14–19 (mild depression); 20–28 (moderate depression); and (29–63) severe depression. Higher total scores indicate more severe depressive symptoms.

Sleep history was assessed at baseline with the 19-item Pittsburgh Sleep Quality Index (PSQI) to assess sleep quality, latency, duration, and disturbances in the past month. A global sleep quality score could range from 0 to 21 and a higher score reflecting more severe sleep disturbance and poor sleep quality. Internal consistency reliability (Cronbach alpha coefficient) was 0.73 in this sample. Current sleep disturbance was assessed using the 21-item General Sleep Disturbance Scale (GSDS). Items on the GSDS assess sleep quality and quantity during the past week on a scale of 0 (not at all) to 7 (every day). Scores can range from 0 to 147 (Lee, 1992). Internal consistency reliability (Cronbach alpha coefficient) for this study was 0.87.

Objective sleep parameters were measured using wrist actigraphy (Ambulatory Monitoring, Inc., Ardsley, NY); a non-invasive watch-like tool that provided sleep-wake patterns via an accelerometer that detected wrist movements of participants over 48 hours at baseline and six weeks after surgery. The actigraph worn by participants' non-dominant wrist detects motion and quantifies the number of movements over a preprogrammed interval (30-second epochs). It has been demonstrated to be reliable and valid with polysomnographic measures of sleep in clinical settings. In surgical patients including women with hysterectomy, in whom traditional sleep monitoring could be difficult, actigraphy would be indicated for characterizing sleep. Wrist actigraphy has accompanying software for an automatic sleep scoring algorithm to allow for quantifying activity and sleep time without bias by researchers, and objectively determines time spent asleep and awake during the night. Sleep parameters of interest included: (a) Total sleep time (TST) in minutes, from the time of 'lights out' to final awakening; (b) sleep efficiency in percentages, of time asleep while in bed; (c) sleep onset latency (SOL) in minutes, between bed time and the first block of inactivity after bed time; (d) awake after sleep onset (WASO) in minutes, awake between sleep onset and wake time; (e) number of awakenings lasting at least 3 minutes; and (f) day time sleep in minutes. A sleep diary was also used for self-monitoring of participant's sleep and daytime activities. Actigraphy data were collected for an average of 3.5 days. Data for each variable was averaged over the recorded time. A sleep diary is useful in conjunction with actigraphy and provides an indication of type of daily activity, including time in bed, trips to the bathroom, or exercise.

3.3. Data analyses

Data were analyzed using descriptive and inferential statistics. Objective sleep data were first downloaded from the actigraph into a personal computer using an interface unit, and then analyzed using Action W4 (Ambulatory Monitoring, Inc., Ardsley, NY) automatic sleep analysis software. Because of a potential 'first-night' adaptation effect, only the second night of sleep data was used for analyses at each time. Pearson product moment correlation coefficients were used to establish significant relationships between the symptom outcome variables (pain, depressed mood and sleep disturbance) and biopsychosocial contextual variables. Multiple regression analyses were performed for those variables with high coefficients ($r > .30$). Repeated measures analysis of variance (RMANOVA) was used to test for within-subject changes in severity of symptom scores from baseline and to test between subjects by type of surgical procedure.

4. Results

Participants ranged in age from 35 to 81 years, with a mean age of 50 (median age 48) ± 10 years. There were 12 Caucasians, 6 African/Black Americans, 4 Asian Americans, and 4 Hispanic women. Over two third of the participants (69%) were employed full-time outside the home, and 77% of them had more than a high school education. Fifteen women were married, six were single, and four were separated or divorced. The majority (73%) had children, and 69% reported a net family annual income of more than $62,000. Time since diagnosis of their disease processes ranged from 1.5 month to 15 years. Four women experienced complications after TAH that included infection, severe leg pain due to thrombosis, or chronic diarrhea.

Descriptive statistics at baseline and six weeks after surgery showed significant changes in their symptom experience. Pain interfered with general activities preoperatively (5.6 ± 1.6) however began to decrease and remain at the lower level by the sixth week (4.7 ± 3.15) after hysterectomy. Eighteen women scored higher means at baseline than postoperatively, indicating that pain had interfered with their general activities; walking, mood, work, sleep, and enjoyment of life before surgery. The Hispanic women perceived significantly higher postoperative pain interference than did the Caucasian women or Black women. The 15 women who had TAH perceived significantly higher pain scores than the 11 women who had LAVH, both before and after surgery ($F = 14.48$, $p < .01$). Women with TAH also scored high on depressed mood than women with LVH after surgery ($F = 4.49$, $p = 0.05$).

Although less than expected, the severity of depressed mood varied greatly in this sample, but averaged 8 ± 2.8 at baseline and decreased to 6 ± 1.71 at six weeks after surgery. Caucasian women (11 ± 3.6) perceived significantly higher depressed mood scores than Hispanic women (8 ± 2.8) pre-operatively ($F = 4.65$, $p = 0.05$). Their scores however reversed at six weeks after surgery, showing that Hispanic women perceived significantly higher depressed mood scores (9 ± 2.8) than Caucasians (5 ± 1.4) or Black Americans (6 ± 1.7). These scores could be arbitrary as they ranged within a minimal depression level that might not be concerns as indicated on BPI.

Furthermore, there was a significant difference in severity of depressed mood perceived by women with TAH and LAVH groups. Women with TAH rated significantly higher scores on a depressed mood inventory than women with LAVH ($F = 4.49$, $p = 0.05$) at six weeks after surgery. For example, although depressed mood scores did not change significantly in women with TAH from the baseline (7.1 ± 1.8) to six weeks after surgery (6.4 ± 2.0), the scores in women with LAVH significantly decreased from the baseline (6.3 ± 1.4) to six weeks after surgery (2.5 ± 0.5) [see TABLE1], showing less severity of depressed mood after surgery. There were no significant differences in symptom severity between women with children and women without children, or between married and single women.

Current sleep disturbance score measured by GSDS in women with TAH averaged 42.1 ± 5.1 at baseline and 38.7 ± 4.9 at six weeks after surgery; and women with LAVH averaged 35 ± 4.1 at baseline and 42.8 ± 5.1 at six weeks after surgery. Women with TAH scored higher on sleep disturbance than women with LAVH at baseline however the scores reversed at six weeks after surgery; women with LAVH scored high on GSDS, indicating that they experienced significantly increased levels of sleep disturbance after surgery.

Latent sleep disturbance scores measured by the Pittsburg sleep quality index (PSQI) in women with TAH and LAVH averaged 7.4 ± 1.1 and 7.6 ± 1.2 respectively at baseline. Compared to the baseline, the average sleep scores of women with TAH (7.5 ± 1.2) and LAVH (7.8 ± 1.3) increased at six weeks after surgery, indicating that their sleep patterns did not improve after surgery over time. Table 1 displays comparison charts of mean differences of pain, depressed mood and sleep disturbance in women with two types of surgical procedures before and six weeks after surgery.

Symptom lists at baseline and 6 weeks after surgery	TAH (n = 15) Mean (SE)	LAVH (n = 11) Mean (SE)
Pain intensity (0-10)		
Baseline	5.6 (2.1)	3.4 (0)
6 weeks after surgery	4.7 (3.6)	3.3 (1)
Beck Depressed Mood (0-63)		
Baseline	7.1 (1.8)	6.3 (1.4)
6 weeks after surgery	6.4 (2.0)	2.5 (0.5)
PSQI-Sleep Disturbance in last week (0-21)		
Baseline	7.4 (1.1)	7.6 (1.2)
6 weeks after surgery	7.5 (1.2)	7.8 (1.3)
GSDS-Sleep Disturbance, current (0-147)		
Baseline	42.1 (5.1)	35 (4.2)
6 weeks after surgery	38.7 (4.9)	42.8 (5.2)

Table 1. Comparison of mean differences of pain, depressed mood, and sleep disturbance in women before and six weeks after total abdominal hysterectomy (TAH) and laparoscopic assisted vaginal hysterectomy (LAVH)

Subjective sleep disturbance was evident at all-time points, with mean PSQI global scores greater than 5, the established cut point for severe sleep disturbance [see TABLE1]. Hispanic and Black women experienced significantly higher PSQI scores than Caucasian or Asian American women at baseline. Similarly, the Black women perceived significantly higher current sleep disturbance on the GSDS than did the Caucasian women at baseline ($F = 8.1$, $p = 0.015$). There were no significant differences in self-reported sleep quality between TAH and LAVH groups.

The sleep actigraphy data are reported on the Table 2 that displays means and standard deviations of sleep data at the baseline and six weeks after surgery. The total sleep time (TST) for the second night of sleep recording at baseline ranged from 301 minutes to 720 minutes with a mean of 392 ± 121 minutes, and number of awakenings ranged from 3 to 21, with a mean of 10 ± 6.0. At six weeks after surgery, the TST ranged from 180 minutes to 540 minutes with a mean of 402 ± 126 minutes. Sleep efficiency decreased from 89% (SD = 8) at the baseline to 82% (SD = 16) at six weeks after surgery. The mean wake after sleep-onset (WASO) increased from 8.48 ± 7.36 minutes to 14.69 ± 12.50 minutes, indicating increase in sleep disturbance. The numbers of awakenings significantly increased from 10 ± 6 at baseline to 20 ± 8 at six weeks after surgery ($F = 2.0$, $p < 0.02$). An additional finding, after surgery, was that the daytime sleep increased to compensate for lack of sleep at night. When actigraphy sleep data were compared by type of surgical procedure, there were no statistically significant differences between TAH and LAVH groups.

Time	Total Sleep Time (minutes)	Sleep Efficiency (%)	Wake After Sleep Onset (minutes)	Number of Awakenings	Sleep Onset Latency (minutes)	Day Sleep (minutes)
Baseline						
Mean	402	89	8.5	10	11.1	3.7
Median	404	91	6.5	8	8.0	3.1
SD	126	8	7.4	6	9.5	2.9
6 weeks Post						
Mean	411	82	14.7	20	13.7	4.0
Median	437	87	11.7	18	6.5	2.7
SD	102	16	12.5	8	2.6	4.1
Significance						
F (*p*)	1.5 (0.12)	0.9 (0.10)	2.1 (0.2)	2.0 (0.02)		

Table 2. Mean Comparisons of sleep efficiency and numbers of awakenings of actigraphy recordings at baseline and six weeks after hysterectomy (n = 26)

Table 3 displays Pearson product moment correlation coefficients of pain, depressed mood, and sleep disturbance symptoms and biopsychosocial variables before and six weeks after surgery. Age was negatively related to current and latent sleep quality, indicating that younger women had more sleep disturbance by self-report. Age was also negatively correlated with pain and depressed mood however the relationship was not statistically significant in this sample.

Preoperative sleep efficiency recorded in wrist actigrpahs was negatively correlated with perceptions of current sleep disturbance of GSDS ($r = -0.51$, $p < 0.01$) and latent sleep disturbance (PSQI) in the past month ($r = -0.64$, $p < 0.01$). Preoperative perception of depressed mood was related with current and latent sleep disturbances ($r = 0.60$, $r = 0.44$, $p < 0.01$). Current sleep disturbance was correlated with the latent sleep disturbance ($r = 0.78$, $p < 0.05$). Postoperative sleep disturbance (PSQI) was also negatively related to age ($r = -0.47$, $p < .002$), and positively correlated with depressed mood ($r = 0.65$, $p < .01$). There were no statistically significant relationships between the pain and other covariables over time in this sample.

Time 1: Baseline	Pittsburg Pain1	Beck Depression1	Current Sleep GSDS1	Latent Sleep Quality PSQI1
Age	-0.45	-0.41	-0.63**	-0.66**
Education level	-0.26	0.10	0.22	0.04
Sleep efficiency	-0.37	-0.04	-0.51*	-0.64**
Pain	1	0.17	0.20	0.27
Depressed mood	0.17	1	0.60*	0.44*
Current sleep disturbance	0.20	0.60*	1	0.78**
Time 2: 6 weeks Post-op	**Pittsburg Pain2**	**Beck Depression2**	**Current Sleep GSDS2**	**Latent Sleep Quality PSQI2**
Age	-0.08	-0.34	-0.45	-0.47*
Education level	-0.48	0.14	0.18	0.24
Sleep efficiency	-0.32	-0.34	-0.39	-0.65**
Pain	1	0.40	0.13	0.17
Depressed Mood	0.40	1	0.65*	0.40
Current sleep disturbance	0.13	0.65*	1	0.57*

Note: * = Correlation is significant at the .05 level (2-tailed); and ** = Correlation is significant at the.01 level (2-tailed)

Table 3. Correlation coefficients between symptom outcome and biopsychosocial variables at baseline (Time 1) and Six Weeks (Time 2) after Surgery

5. Discussion

This study examines key symptoms of pain, depressed mood and disturbed sleep experienced by culturally diverse women who have undergone total abdominal hysterectomy (TAH) and laparoscopic assisted vaginal hysterectomy (LAVH); and evaluates their biopsychosocial variables in relation to the symptoms preoperatively and six weeks after surgery. Results indicate that women experience high levels of pain that interfere with their daily activities prior to surgery. Findings also suggest that women who undergo TAH perceive significantly higher pain scores than the women who receive LAVH postoperatively. Pain severity, however, is not correlated with any other variables.

The severity of depressed mood varies greatly in this sample. Women with TAH score higher on depressed mood than women with LAVH before and after surgery. In this study, women's depressive symptoms improved after surgery, especially in women with LAVH. Although Caucasian women experienced worsen symptoms of depressed mood than Hispanic women at baseline, their scores reversed after surgery, with improved perception of depressed mood, while Hispanic women reported worsening mood. This outcome coincides with the study conducted by Gibson, Joffe, and Bromberger's [45] in that the researchers found women who had a hysterectomy with or without bilateral oophorectomy in midlife did not experience more negative mood symptoms in the years after surgery; however they reported that women's depressive and anxiety symptoms improved over the course of the menopausal transition. Similarly, in their review, Darwish, Atlantis, and Mohamed-Taysir [46] claimed that hysterectomy was associated with a decreased risk of clinically relevant depression and standardized depression outcomes. However Wang and colleagues [21] argued that their patients had obvious depression and anxiety symptoms before and after hysterectomy; and those who received psychological interventions decreased the depression scores significantly. Interestingly, Gómez-Campelo, Bragado-Álvarez, and Hernández-Lloreda [47] identified psychological distress of women that had undergone hysterectomy and mastectomy; and found both surgeries caused body image disturbance and depression for women. It appears that women might feel depressed when they have lost a part of their womanhood after hysterectomy, however understanding the need, risks, and benefits of surgery would help alleviate depressive feelings. Based on a current findings, hysterectomy alone does not have a physical basis for resulting in depression; therefore women can prevent this symptom by thoroughly understanding the surgical cases.

Women also report significant levels of subjective and objective sleep disturbances before and after surgery. Although the subjective sleep disturbance is significantly greater in Black and Hispanic women at baseline, there is no statistically significant ethnic difference in objective data measured by actigraphy recordings in this study.

Use of a wrist actigraph for measuring objective sleep data provides the changing pattern of sleep over time. Compared to the preoperative actigraphy data, women experience a progressive decrease in sleep efficiency and increase in day time sleep and numbers of awakenings during nights at six weeks after surgery. Sleep efficiency is negatively correlated with perceptions of current and latent sleep disturbance. This is a concern that healthcare providers should be aware as women might develop further risks and other complications if the sleep disturbance continues after surgery.

Preoperative and postoperative sleep disturbances are negatively related to age, indicating that younger women experience worse sleep disturbance; and positively correlated with depressed mood. It is worthy to note that certain correlations may exist between the physiological and psychological outcomes of hysterectomy. For instance, symptoms such as preoperative depressive moods may increase pain thresholds that may eventually cause poor sleep after hysterectomy. It is well known that signs of depressive mood may include insomnia and restlessness. Therefore, depressive mood may partially account for sleep disturbance after hysterectomy. Further research on the correlations between the physiological, psychological, demographic, and social factors would contribute in developing an integrated and comprehensive nursing care plan for women with hysterectomy.

6. Conclusion

This study examines symptoms of pain, depressed mood and sleep disturbance of women that have undergone abdominal and vaginal hysterectomy using subjective and objective measurements. Without complications, most women with a vaginal hysterectomy recover within a few weeks however those who undergo an abdominal hysterectomy may require six to eight weeks to recover and return to normal routines. Therefore, it is important for women to understand the possible risks involved with both types of surgery prior to having one.

The study provides important findings that women experience before and after hysterectomy and documents symptom severity and related biopsychosocial variables. Although the severity of pain and depressed mood decreased, women continue to experience poor sleep six weeks after surgery. With a small sample, results are difficult to generalize to the large population of women before and after hysterectomy. However, significant findings of the study allow for healthcare professionals in developing and implementing potential interventions that may benefit women considering the procedures.

Acknowledgements

This research was supported by grants from the American Nurses' Foundation and National Institute of Nursing Research (T32NR07088).

Author details

Kimberly H. Kim

Address all correspondence to: Kimberly.kim@csueastbay.edu

California State University, East Bay, Hayward, CA, USA

References

[1] Brandsborg B, Nikolajsen L, Kehlet H, Jensen T. Chronic pain after hysterectomy. Acta Anaesthesiologica Scandinavica. 2008; 52(3): 327-331.

[2] Cohen S, Hollingsworth A, Rubin M, Graff B, Thomas J, Welz H, Wehry L. Psychosocial adaptation during recovery from hysterectomy. WebmedCentral Obstetrics and Gynecology. 2011; 2(3): WMC001660. http://www.webmedcentral.com/wmcpdf/Article_WMC001660.pdf

[3] Cohen SL, Vitonis A, Einarsson J. Updated hysterectomy surveillance and factors associated with minimally invasive hysterectomy. Journal of the Society of Laparoscopic Surgeries. 2014; 18(3): DOI: 10.4293/JSLS.2014.00096

[4] Pinto P, McIntyre T, Almeida A, Araújo-Soares V. The mediating role of pain catastrophizing in the relationship between presurgical anxiety and acute postsurgical pain after hysterectomy. Pain. 2012; 153(1): 218–226.

[5] Chen I, Lisonkova S, Allaire C, Williams C, Yong P, Joseph KS. Routes of hysterectomy in women with benign uterine disease in the Vancouver coastal health and providence health care regions: A retrospective cohort analysis. CMAJ Open. 2014; 2(4): E273–E280. DOI: 10.9778/cmajo.20130080

[6] Laberge PY, Singh SS. Surgical approach to hysterectomy: Introducing the concept of technicity. Journal of Obstetrics Gynecology Canada. 2009; 31: 1050-1053.

[7] Kim K, Lee K. Sleep and fatigue symptoms in women before and 6 weeks after hysterectomy. Journal of Obstetric, Gynecologic & Neonatal Nursing. 2009; 38(3): 344-352.

[8] Mahnert N, Morgan D, Campbell D, Johnston C, As-Sanie S. Unexpected Gynecologic Malignancy Diagnosed After Hysterectomy Performed for Benign Indications. Obstetrics and Gynecology. Feb 2015; 125(2):397-405. doi: 10.1097/AOG.0000000000000642.

[9] Wise LA, Li Se, Palmer JR, Rosenberg L. Depressive symptoms and risk of uterine leiomyomata. Am J Obstet Gynecol. Dec 13 2014; pii: S0002-9378(14)02436-3. DOI: 10.1016/j.ajog.2014.12.012.

[10] Bayram G, Beji N. Psychosexual adaptation and quality of life after hysterectomy. Sexuality and Disability. 2010; 28(1): 3-13.

[11] Peterson Z, Rothenberg J, Bilbrey S, Heiman J. Sexual functioning following elective hysterectomy: The role of surgical and psychosocial variables. Journal of Sex Research. 2010; 47(6): 513-527.

[12] Poliquin V, Victory R, Vilos GA. Epidemiology, presentation, and management of retroperitoneal leiomyomata: systematic literature review and case report. Journal of Minimally Invasive Gynecology. 2008; 15(2): 152-160.

[13] Kovac SR. Clinical opinion: Guidelines for hysterectomy. American Journal of Obstetric and Gynecology. 2004; 191(2): 635-640.

[14] Pitter MC, Simmonds C, Seshadri-Kreaden U, Hubert HB. The impact of different surgical modalities for hysterectomy on satisfaction and patient reported outcomes. Interactive Journal of Medical Research. 2014; 3(3): e11. DOI: 10.2196/ijmr.3160.

[15] Wilcox L, Koonin L, Pokras R, Strauss L, Xia Z, Peterson H. Hysterectomy in the United States. 1988-1990. Obstetrics & Gynecology. 1994; 83(4): 549-555.

[16] Li G, Yan X, Shang H, Wang G, Chen L, Han Y. A comparison of laparoscopic radical hysterectomy and pelvic lymphadenectomy and laparotomy in the treatment of Ib-IIa cervical cancer. Gynecological Oncology. 2007; 105(1): 176-180.

[17] Susini T, Massi G, Amunni G, Carroerp C, Marchionni M, Taddei G, Scarselli G. Vaginal hysterectomy and abdominal hysterectomy for treatment of endometrial cancer in the elderly. Gynecological Oncology. 2005; 96(2): 362-367.

[18] Boggess JF, Gehrig PA, Cantrell L. A comparative study of 3 surgical methods for hysterectomy with staging for endometrial cancer: robotic assistance, laparoscopy, laparotomy. American Journal of Obstetrics Gynecology. 2008; 199(4): 360.e1–360.e9.

[19] Hopkins M, Richmond A, Cheng G, Davidson S, Spillman M, Sheeder J. Lymphovascular space invasion in robotic surgery for endometrial cancer. Journal of the Society of Laparoendoscopic Surgeons. 2014; 18(3): doi: 10.4293/JSLS.2014.00021

[20] Sehlo M, Ramadani, H. Depression following hysterectomy. Current Psychiatry.2010; 17(2): 1-6.

[21] Wang F, Li CB, Li S, Li Q. Integrated interventions for improving negative emotions and stress reactions of young women receiving total hysterectomy. International Journal of Clinical and Experimental Medicine. 2014; 7(1): 331-316.

[22] Barranger E, Isnard F, Bricou A, Darai E, Delpech Y. Quality of life after laparoscopic radical hysterectomy for cervical cancer: Study of 22 cases. Gynecologic Obstetric Fertility. 2012; 40(10) 572-577.

[23] Lamvu G. Role of hysterectomy in the treatment of chronic pelvic pain. Obstetrics & Gynecology.2011; 117(5): 1175-1178.

[24] Aerts L, Enzlin P, Verhaeghe J, Poppe W, Vergote I, Amant F. Sexual function in women after surgical treatment for endometrial cancer: A prospective controlled study, The Journal of Sexual Medicine. 2014; doi: 10.1111/jsm.12764.

[25] Keskin G, Gumus A. Turkish hysterectomy and mastectomy patients - depression, body image, sexual problems and spouse relationships. Asian Pacific Journal of Cancer Prevention. 2011; 12: 425-432.

[26] Andersen LL, Ottesen B, Alling Møller LM, Gluud C, Tabor A, Zobbe V. Subtotal versus total abdominal hysterectomy: randomized clinical trial with 14-year questionnaire follow-up. American Journal of Obstetrics and Gynecology. 2014; pii: S0002-9378(14)02498-3. DOI: 10.1016/j.ajog.2014.12.039.

[27] Tom S, Kuh D, Guralnik J, Mishra G. Self-reported sleep difficulty during the menopausal transition: results from a prospective cohort study. 2010; Menopause, 17(6): 1128-1135.

[28] Sheizaf B, Almog B, Salamah K, Shehata F, Takefman J, Tulandi T. A pragmatic evaluation of sleep patterns before gynecologic surgery. Gynecological Surgery. 2011; 8(2): 151-155.

[29] Ouladsahebmadarek E, Sayyah-Melli M, Jafari M, Gojazadeh M, Khaki A. Hysterectomy versus GnRH agonist for dysfunctional uterine bleeding in premenopausal women. African Journal of Pharmacy and Pharmacology. 2011; 5(12): 1547-1552.

[30] Solnik MJ, Munro MG. Indications and alternatives to hysterectomy. Clinical Obstetrics and Gynecology.2014; 57(1): 14-42.

[31] Tiwana KK, Nibhoria S, Monga T, Phutela R. Histopathological audit of 373 non- oncological hysterectomies in a teaching hospital. Pathology Research International, 2014; DOI: 10.1155/2014/468715.

[32] Stovall TG, Ling FW, Crawford DA. Hysterectomy for chronic pelvic pain of presumed uterine etiology. Obstet Gynecol. 1990 Apr; 75(4):676-9.

[33] Darnall B, Li H. Hysterectomy and predictors for opioid prescription in a chronic pain clinic sample. Pain Medicine. 2011; 12(2): 196-203.

[34] Farquhar C, Sadler L, Stewart A. A prospective study of outcomes five years after hysterectomy in premenopausal women. Australian & New Zealand Journal of Obstetrics Gynaecology. 2008; 48(5): 510-516.

[35] Vercellini P, Viganó P, Somigliana E, Abbiati A, Barbara G, Fedele L. Medical, surgical and alternative treatments for chronic pelvic pain in women: a descriptive review. Gynecological Endocrinology. 2009; 25(4): 208–221.

[36] Pokkinen SM, Kalliomäki ML, Yli-Hankala A, Nieminen K. Less post-operative pain after laparoscopic hysterectomy than after vaginal hysterectomy. Archives of Gynecology and Obstetrics. 2014 Dec 31; [Epub ahead of print]

[37] Heliövaara-Peippo S, Halmesmäki K, Hurskainen R, Teperi J, Grenman S, Kivelä A, Kujansuu E, Tuppurainen M, Vuorma S, Yliskoski M, Paavonen J. The effect of hysterectomy or levonorgestrel-releasing intrauterine system on lower abdominal pain and back pain among women treated for menorrhagia: a five-year randomized controlled trial. Acta Obstetricia et Gynecologica Scandinavica. 2009; 88(12): 1389-1396.

[38] Gibson C, Bromberger J, Weiss G, Thurston R, Sowers M, Matthews K. Negative attitudes and affect do not predict elective hysterectomy: a prospective analysis from the Study of Women's Health Across the Nation. Menopause.2011; 18(5): 499-507.

[39] Ewalds-Kvist S, Hirvonen T, Kvist M, Lertola K, Niemelä P. Depression, anxiety, hostility and hysterectomy. Journal of Psychosomatic Obstetrics & Gynecology. 2005; 26(3): 193-204.

[40] Cooper R, Mishra G, Hardy R, and Kuh D. Hysterectomy and subsequent psychological health: Findings from a British birth cohort study. Journal of Affective Disorders. 2009; 115(1): 122-130.

[41] Vandyk A, Brenner I, Tranmer J, Kerkhof E. Depressive symptoms before and after elective hysterectomy. Journal of Obstetric, Gynecologic & Neonatal Nursing. 2011; 40(5): 566-576.

[42] Mantani A, Yamashita H, Fujikawa T, Yamawaki S. Higher incidence of hysterectomy and oophorectomy in women suffering from clinical depression: Retrospective chart review. Psychiatry & Clinical Neurosciences. 2010; 64(1): 95-98.

[43] Wang X, Lambert C, Lambert V. Anxiety, depression and coping strategies in post-hysterectomy Chinese women prior to discharge. International Nursing Review. 2007; 54(3): 271-279.

[44] Lee K. Self- reported sleep disturbance in employed women. Sleep. 1992;15: 493-498.

[45] Gibson C, Joffe H, Bromberger J, Thurston R, Lewis T. Mood symptoms after natural menopause and hysterectomy with and without bilateral oophorectomy among women in midlife. Obstetrics Gynecology. 2013; 119(5): 935-941.

[46] Darwish M, Atlantis E, Mohamed-Taysir T. Psychological outcomes after hysterectomy for benign conditions: a systematic review and meta-analysis. European Journal of Obstetrics, Gynecology, and Reproductive Biology. 2014; 174: 5-19.

[47] Gómez-Campelo P, Bragado-Álvarez C, Hernández-Lloreda MJ. Psychological distress in women with breast and gynecological cancer treated with radical surgery. Psychooncology. 2014 Apr; 23(4):459-66.

[48] Brooks SE, Mullins CD, Guo C, Chen TT, Gardner JF, Baquet CR. Resource utilization for patients undergoing hysterectomy with or without lymph node dissection for endometrial cancer. Gynecol Oncol. 2002 May; 85(2):242-9.

Section 2

Alternatives to Hysterectomy for Uterine Myomas

Chapter 2

Laparoscopic Transient Uterine Artery Occlusion and Myomectomy for Symptomatic Uterine Myoma as an Alternative to Hysterectomy

Yanzhou Wang, Li Deng, Huicheng Xu,
Yong Chen and Zhiqing Liang

Additional information is available at the end of the chapter

Abstract

Objective: To compare the clinical outcomes of laparoscopic transient uterine artery ligation plus myomectomy (LTUAL) to simple laparoscopic myomectomy (LM) for symptomatic myomas.

Methods: A comparative observational study was adopted; 167 patients with a diagnosis of symptomatic uterine myoma were retrospectively observed. And 84 patients underwent LTUAL and LM, 83 patients underwent LM only. Operative time, blood loss, gonadal hormone level, uterine artery resistance index, menorrhea, pregnancy rate, and recurrence rate of myoma were evaluated.

Results: The intraoperative blood loss in the LTUAL group was lower than in the LM group. The menstrual blood volume (MBV) and the menstrual period of the LTUAO group were unchanged after operation relative to the prediseased volume. No significant difference was found in the resistance index of the uterine artery blood flow, the recurrence rate, and the fertility rate between the LTUAL and the LM groups.

Conclusions: LTUAL and LM are a promising surgical treatment for symptomatic uterine myoma and did not produce any appreciable adverse effect on fertility.

Keywords: Laparoscopic, Uterine artery occlusion, Myomectomy, Uterine myoma

INTECH
open science | open minds

© 2015 The Author(s). Licensee InTech. This chapter is distributed under the terms of the Creative Commons Attribution License (http://creativecommons.org/licenses/by/3.0), which permits unrestricted use, distribution, and reproduction in any medium, provided the original work is properly cited.

1. Introduction

Uterine myomas are the most common benign tumor of the female reproductive system. It is estimated that they occur in up to 35% of women 35 years of age [1]. Most of these myomas are asymptomatic, although some may cause symptoms that require a definite treatment. Approximately 30% of women with myomas have been reported to have menstrual abnormalities, most often menorrhagia. Dysmenorrhea also may occur. Acute pain can occur with red degeneration, necrosis, and torsion of a pedunculated myoma. Large myomas can also stimulate urinary tract compression, resulting in symptoms such as urinary frequency and urgency. Myomas may also cause infertility and miscarriage [2].

There are many therapeutic strategies, but the management of women with symptomatic uterine myomas depends on the patient's age, the reasons for treatment, the issue of fertility preservation, and the patient's preference. Although hysterectomy has long been considered a good choice if women have completed childbearing, there are many other therapeutic approaches available for preservation of the uterus, because psychologically, the uterus has been regarded as the regulator and controller of important physiologic functions, a sexual organ, a source of energy and vitality, and a maintainer of youth and attractiveness. Some of these therapies include uterine artery embolization (UAE), MRgFUS (magnetic resonance-guided focused ultrasound surgery), and ultrasound-guided ablation (VizAblate™ [Gynesonics, Redwood City, CA, USA] and Acessa™ [Halt Medical, Inc., Brentwood, CA, USA] procedures). The standard treatment for symptomatic uterine fibroids has always been myomectomy. Myomectomy has been traditionally performed by laparotomy, but over the past decade, laparoscopic and hysteroscopic techniques have been developed. The surgery can now be performed laparoscopically and hysteroscopically. Laparoscopic surgery has seen significant improvement in its techniques and instruments, and has been developed and used in the management of various kinds of benign diseases. Although some concerns about the role of laparoscopic myomectomy (LM) as a treatment option for symptomatic uterine myomas are still present, it is still widely used for symptomatic subserosal fibroids and can even be used for intramural fibroids, depending on the position of the fibroid and the skills of the surgeon. Many comparison studies have evaluated the safety and feasibility of abdominal myomectomy and LM [3]. These studies showed that LM is clearly associated with shorter hospitalization, faster recovery, less expense, less pain, less blood loss, less fever, and fewer surgical complications compared with abdominal myomectomy. Pregnancy rates and recurrence rates appear to be comparable between LM and abdominal myomectomy [3]. Therefore, the use of LM can be considered as one of the choices in the management of women with symptomatic uterine myomas.

Myomectomy is a challenging procedure for gynecologists and can result in excessive blood loss. In general, it is suitable only for patients who have a few relatively small myomas or myomas that are primarily below the serosa [4]. The relative contraindications of LM include a history of multiple, large, intrauterine wall myomas [5]. With recent technique advances, LM can be performed as the treatment for relatively large uterine fibroids. However, the challenges of increased operation time and the high risk of blood loss still remain [6]. Several methods to control blood loss during LM are available, including the use of dilute vasopressin, hypotensive anesthesia, and administration of GnRH agonists. Until now, there is no single method to completely control intraoperative blood loss and prevent postoperative exudation from the uterine incisional wound.

Recently, a major development in overcoming this problem is the laparoscopic uterine artery occlusion (LUAO) [7], which was introduced in 2001. This procedure can result in remarkably decreased blood loss in LM [8], and it has expanded the application of LM greatly, such as the large, multiple, and deep myomas located in the uterus. However, the possible side effects of LUAO, such as the increased abortion rate and preterm delivery [9, 10], lack further verification in literature. As a result, we have developed a new approach to LUAO: laparoscopic transient uterine artery ligation (LTUAL). In this study, we attempt to elucidate this new approach and evaluate the possible results of LTUAL and LM on outcomes such as ovary function, recurrence rates, and fertility compared with traditional LM.

2. Materials and methods

2.1. Patients

A comparative observational study was adopted. Between January 1, 2006, and June 31, 2008, 167 patients with a diagnosis of symptomatic uterine myoma and who were hospitalized at Southwest Hospital in Chongqing, China, for LM were enrolled in this study.

Per the inclusion criteria, all patients had symptoms attributable to myomas, including menorrhagia, bulge sensation, pain, and urinary frequency, with the most common being menorrhagia. The diagnosis was confirmed by ultrasonography or computed tomography scan. All the patients preferred not to undergo a hysterectomy. The exclusion criteria eliminated women who were older than 43 years or had an additional gynecologic disease such as adenomyoma, genital malignant tumor, genital malformation, premature ovarian failure, polycystic ovary, fallopian tubes adhesion or imperforation, or sactosalpinx. Women whose husbands had abnormal results of the seminal fluid test were also excluded.

The institutional review board of our institution approved the study, and all participants provided written informed consent before entry. All patients in this study were thoroughly notified of the benefits, curative effects, potential risks, and uncertain fertility issues related to uterine artery occlusion. Eighty-four patients who accepted LTUAL were placed in the LTUAL group and treated with LTUAL and LM. Eighty-four patients who refused LTUAL were placed in the LM group and received LM only. There was no difference in the age, the body mass index, the maximal diameter, and the location and number of myomas between the two groups (Table 1).

Characteristic	LTUAL (n = 84)	LM (n = 83)	*P value*
Age, y	32.5 (25–43)	32 (26–43)	0.936
Body mass index, kg/m^2	22.65 (18.1–27.7)	23.1 (18.4–27.1)	0.927
Pregnancy history, n			
Nullipara	52 (61.9%)	59 (71.1%)	
Multipara	32 (38.1%)	24 (28.9%)	
Symptoms, n			
Menorrhagia	61 (72.6%)	56 (67.5%)	0.468
Bulge sensation	52 (61.9%)	48 (57.8%)	0.591
Pain	19 (22.6%)	30 (36.1%)	0.055
Urinary frequency	16 (19.0%)	21 (25.3%)	0.331
Myomas			
Diameter, cm	5.8 (3–12)	5.9 (3–11)	0.504
Location, n			0.973
Subserous	22 (26.2%)	20 (24.1%)	
Intrauterine wall	32 (38.1%)	28 (33.7%)	
Submucosal, n	7 (8.3%)	9 (10.8%)	
Multiple, n	23 (27.4%)	26 (31.3%)	
Average multiple number	4 (2–13)	3.5 (2–8)	0.87

Table 1. Basic characteristics of the enrolled women.

2.2. Operative procedures

All procedures were performed under general endotracheal anesthesia. The LTUAL technique was performed like the LUAO previously described [7], except that the uterine artery was transiently ligated by a slipknot with a surgical silk suture. The successful artery ligation could be confirmed as previously described [8]. Next, the LM progress was performed as previously described [8]. Last, the slipknot was removed and the uterine arteries were recanalized. Finally, the fallopian tube perfusion test was performed to exclude patients with broken uterine walls or obstructed fallopian tubes. Blood loss was estimated by calculating the blood volume of the suction machine during surgery.

2.3. Follow-up method

The follow-up time ranged 10–40 months. The routine time of interview was 3 and 6 months and at 1, 2, and 3 years after the operation or at any time if any problems arose. All patients were advised to engage in contraceptive measures by the use of condoms for 24 months. After this period, women were free to seek conception.

2.4. Assessment of menstrual patterns

To evaluate the effect of LTUAL on menorrhea, a questionnaire was sent to each of the patients when compiling their case history. The number of menstrual pads used by each woman was recorded during three menstrual cycles: before the diseased state, during the disease, and after surgery. We set a value of 1 for the menstrual blood volume (MBV) index for the prediseased period for each patient. The diseased MBV index is equal to the number of menstrual pads used during the diseased period divided by the number of menstrual pads used before the diseased period. Once regular menorrhea recovered at least for 6 months following the operation, the postoperation MBV index was recorded as the diseased MBV index. Because the MBV during the diseased state was mostly irregularly increased in the presence of myomas and was inconsequential for the evaluation of the single effect of LTUAL, we decided to abandon this index. The only comparison was made for the two periods: before the disease occurred and postoperation.

2.5. Recurrence assessment

All patients received an ultrasound examination 3 months after the operation to confirm the effectiveness of the procedure and to exclude the patients with residual myomas; they also received an ultrasound examination at each routine interview. The recurrence was defined when uterine myomas, with a minimum diameter of 0.5 cm, were found in patients without residual myomas.

2.6. Statistical analysis

SPSS 11.5 (SPSS, Inc., Chicago, IL) was used for statistical analysis. Data are presented as mean ± SD, number (%), and median (range). The difference in means between the groups was tested by using an ANOVA test, if the variable under comparison was not normally distributed. The rank sum test was used. The categorical variables are presented as percentages, and were compared using χ^2 tests or Fisher's exact tests. $P<0.05$ was considered statistically significant.

3. Results

All 167 patients underwent laparoscopic operations successfully without intraoperative complications, with no cases converting to laparotomy. In the LM group, one patient experienced a 4-hour operation and lost 600 ml of blood during surgery, which necessitated a blood transfusion; later, a wound infection developed, and the patient stayed in the hospital for 21 days for intravenous fluid and antibiotic therapy. Five patients in the LM group received blood transfusions during or after the operation. Two patients in the LTUAL group and four patients in the LM group suffered from urinary tract infections. In addition, one patient in the LTUAL group and four patients in the LM group had a high fever (body temperature > 38.5°C) for more than 3 days and stayed in the hospital for antibiotic therapy for 1 week. There were no severe complications such as ureter, bladder, or bowel injury during the perioperative period. All pathologic examinations documented the presence of uterine leiomyomas. There was no statistical difference in the average operation time between the LTUAL and the LM groups (*P*=0.41). The transient ligation time in the LTUAL group ranged 55–155 minutes, and the median time was 98.5 minutes. Blood loss was significantly lower in the LTUAL group than in the LM group (*P*<0.01). The mean postoperative hospital stay was 3.8 days (range, 3–21 days).

The results of the menorrhea assessment are given in Table 2. The MBV, menstrual period, and menstrual cycle were unchanged after surgery in the two groups compared with before the disease occurred (*P*>0.05).

	LTUAL	LM
Volume rank (before disease)	1.00 ± 0.00	1.00 ± 0.00
Volume rank (after surgery)	1.00 ± 0.00	1.00 ± 0.10
P	0.071	0.316
Menstrual period (before disease)	5 ± 1	5 ± 1
Menstrual period (after surgery)	5 ± 1	5 ± 1
P	0.227	0.091
Menstrual cycle (before disease)	28 ± 2	29 ± 3
Menstrual cycle (after surgery)	28.5 ± 2	29 ± 2
P	0.782	0.326

Table 2. Menorrhea evaluation (median ± interquartile range).

The uterine artery resistance index (RI) was also tested. There was no statistical difference found between the two groups each time, at the preoperative period, and at 3 days, 6 months, and 12 months after surgery in each group (*P*>0.05; Table 3).

Period	LTUAL (n = 84)	LM (n = 83)	*P value*
Before surgery	0.73 (0.48–0.90)	0.71 (0.50–0.88)	0.156
After surgery			
3 days	0.705 (0.49–0.87)	0.69 (0.53–0.89)	0.744
6 months	0.69 (0.48–0.89)	0.695 (0.47–0.88)	0.466
12 months	0.69 (0.48–0.87)	0.70 (0.49–0.86)	0.882

Table 3. Comparison of uterine artery resistance index.

Recurrence rates following the different procedures were examined next. There were six cases confirmed with residual myomas by ultrasonography 3 days after the operations, and these cases were excluded from those subjected to recurrence follow-up for the interference of the recurrence assessment. The data from the remaining the cases were collected and are presented in Table 4. There was no statistical difference between the LTUAL group and the LM group (*P*=0.237).

The fertility evaluation is presented in Table 4. In the LTUAL group, 31 patients were still using contraception at the 2-year follow-up, and five of the remaining 53 patients have consistently used contraception 2 years later. In the remaining 48 patients seeking pregnancy, the outcomes were as follows: one patient had an ectopic pregnancy that was later subjected to treatment by methotrexate; 15 patients conceived normally, and of these, 9 patients proceeded to full-term pregnancy. In the LM group, 28 patients were still using contraception at the 2-year follow up; 13 patients were currently still using contraception 2 years later. Among the remaining 42 patients attempting to become pregnant, miscarriage occurred in two patients and 16 patients had a normal pregnancy (Table 4), half of whom carried a baby to full-term. There was no statistical difference between the LTUAL and the LM groups (*P*=0.495).

	LTUAL (n = 84)	LM (n = 83)	*P value*	OR (95% CI)
Operation duration, min	121.92 ± 18.48[a]	126.33 ± 27.13	0.313	—
Blood loss, ml[b]	75 (40–190)	170 (100–600)	0.001	—
Recurrence, n	16/82 (19.51%)[c]	10/79 (12.66%)[c]	0.237	1.673 (0.708–3.950)
Pregnancy, n	15/48 (31.25%)[d]	16/42 (38.10%)[d]	0.495	0.739 (0.309–1.767)

Note: OR = odds ratio; CI = confidence interval.

[a] Mean ± SD.

[b] Precise scale = 5 ml.

[c] Patients with residual myomas were excluded.

[d] Patients still using contraception were excluded. Total number of women included those who were no longer using contraception and were seeking pregnancy.

Table 4. Surgical parameters and recurrence, pregnancy follow-up data.

4. Discussion

During LM, failure of hemostasis is the primary factor resulting in conversion to laparotomy [11]. However, this problem was addressed by the introduction of LUAO: Liu et al. [7] reported LUAO as a new method for treating symptomatic myomas, but they used this technique as a primary treatment without proceeding to myomectomy, and the recurrence rate was reported as 28.4% within the 4-year follow-up period [12]. In our previous study [8], this technique was used as a supplement for LM first, with the uterine arteries being blocked while the myomas were completely removed. This technique resulted in a remarkable blood loss in the operation and a low recurrence rate, but possible side effects in uterine or ovarian function, especially long-term effects on fertility, need further study.

Because of the possible side effects of LUAO on fertility [9, 10], we developed LTUAL to be used in patients who wish to comply after a thorough explanation of the pros and cons of the procedure. This discussion allowed for the evaluation of the effects of LTUAL on menorrhea, fertility, and the recurrence rates of myomas.

In this study, LTUAL decreased intraoperative blood loss remarkably compared with LM. With the critical problem being tackled, we were able to conduct LM for large, multiple, intrauterine wall and especially submucosal myomas. There was no difference in the duration of the operation between the two groups, because in our experience, LTUAL can be performed within 10 minutes by an experienced gynecologist. However, in the LM group, more time is usually spent trying to maintain the hemostasis of the sutured wounds of the uterine cavity.

A problem related to this study may be the ligation time of the uterine artery. Traditional uterine tourniquets are usually best used for no more than 1 hour [13] to avoid irreversible damage to the uterine myometrium and the risk of embolic events. Although a review showed no embolic phenomena after detorsion in ischemic necrotic twisted adnexa [14], Wang et al. [15] used average occlusion periods of approximately 2 hours without any complications. Our experience would suggest that the occlusion period of the uterine arteries is not a considerable problem because of the intact ovarian and vaginal ascending arteries, which compose part of the triple-extrinsic uterine blood supply system. At the least, our transient ligation period (97.93 ± 19.08 minutes) was verified to be harmless to the myometrium and did not induce any complications.

By the assessment of unchanged uterine RI, menstrual pattern, and the recurrence of myomas, we thought the LTUAL interfered minimally with ovary function, uterine myometrium, and the uterus status, which were important for fertility.

Because of deficiencies associated with our laboratory, we had to study ovarian function indirectly by the indices of uterine artery RI and the menorrhea change. First, the blood supply of the ovary is the main factor that influences ovarian function. In this type of surgery, the ovarian vessels were untouched; the only operation that could disturb the ovarian blood supply was the LTUAL, because the uterine artery is one of the ramus anastomoticus of ovarian blood supply. We found no differences of the uterine artery RI between the two groups and between different periods. As a result, we verified that the blood supply in the ovaries was not disturbed by LTUAL. Second, no differences in menorrhea were found between the prediseased state and the postoperative state in the LTUAL and LM groups, so we inferred that LTUAL had minimal interference on ovary function. In our previous study [8] and in the recent literature [12, 16, 17], the recurrence rate using LUAO was low and markedly lower than that reported for abdominal myomectomy and LM [18, 19, 20]. The decreased blood supply to the uterus induced gradual necrosis of the myomas. Lee et al. [21] found a markedly decreased RI index 4 months after LUAO compared with that before surgery. Other similar researches [22, 23] found a shrinking of myomas after LUAO and confirmed that apoptosis was the primary mechanism by which this occurred [23]. In contrast, the recurrence rates appear to be no different between the LTUAL and the LM groups. Thus, minimal interference of LTUAL on the uterine artery and uterine status is confirmed by unchanged menorrhea and recurrence rate of myomas.

In this study, the gestation rate of patients was evaluated over a 16–36 months follow-up. No difference was found between the LTUAL and the LM groups on the gestation rate, and some patients gave birth to full-term babies; therefore, there is no statistical proof that the LTUAL has any side effect on fertility.

Moreover, the reduced adhesion formation following laparoscopy is another benefit for fertility of these patients. For laparotomy, the postoperative rate of adhesions, which are the most probable risk for infertility, is high (80%) [24]. It has been hypothesized that laparoscopic surgery, by maintaining hemostasis and minimizing peritoneal trauma and inflammation [25], may result in reduced adhesion formation following abdominal and pelvic surgery [26-29]. This lack of adhesions could theoretically help to diminish the risk of infertility. Therefore, we consider LTUAL to be a promising method in patients who wish to preserve fertility.

5. Conclusion

LTUAL preceded by LM provides several benefits to patients and is more in accordance with the modern medical opinion regarding the preservation of the uterus and with limited side effects on ovarian function and fertility. In addition, the procedure is preferable in patients who wish to undergo future pregnancies. However, LTUAL plus LM cannot decrease the recurrence rate of myomas. It must be emphasized that this study was limited by the lack of randomization, and on the basis of this a more rigorous and detailed study should be undertaken. We strongly suggest that a randomized controlled trial is a next step for further verification and discussion.

Nomenclature

LM; laparoscopic myomectomy

LUAO; laparoscopic uterine artery occlusion

LTUAL; laparoscopic transient uterine artery ligation

MBV; menstrual blood volume

Author details

Yanzhou Wang, Li Deng, Huicheng Xu, Yong Chen and Zhiqing Liang*

*Address all correspondence to: zhi.lzliang@gmail.com

Department of Obstetrics and Gynecology, Southwest Hospital, Third Military Medical University, Chongqing, People's Republic of China

References

[1] Dixon D, Parrott EC, Segars JH, Olden K, Pinn VW. The Second National Institutes of Health International Congress on advances in uterine leiomyoma research: conference summary and future recommendations. Fertil Steril 2006;86:800–6.

[2] Munro MG, Brill AI. Gynecologic endoscopy. In: Berek JS, Hillard PJA, Adashi EY, eds. Novak's Gynecology. 13th ed. Baltimore: Lippincott Williams and Wilkins, 2002:714.

[3] Hurst BS, Matthews ML, Marshburn PB. Laparoscopic myomectomy for symptomatic uterine myomas. Fertil Steril 2005;83:1–23.

[4] Seracchioli R, Rossi S, Govoni F, Rossi E, Venturoli S, Bulletti C, et al. Fertility and obstetric outcome after laparoscopic myomectomy of large myomata: a randomised comparison with abdominal myomectomy. Hum Reprod 2000;15:2663–8.

[5] Daniel JF, Gurtey LD. Laparoscopic treatment of clinically significant symptomatic uterine myomas. J Gynecol Surg 1991;7:37.

[6] Wang CJ, Yuen LT, Lee CL, Kay N, Soong YK. Laparoscopic myomectomy for large uterine fibroids: a comparative study. Surg Endosc 2006;20:1427–30.

[7] Liu WM, Ng HT, Wu YC, Yen YK, Yuan CC. Laparoscopic bipolar coagulation of uterine vessels: a new method for treating symptomatic myomas. Fertil Steril 2001;75:417–22.

[8] Liang Z, Xu H, Chen Y, Li Y, Zhang Q. Laparoscopic blockage of uterine artery and myomectomy: a new method of treating symptomatic uterine leiomyomas. Surg Endosc 2006;20:983–6.

[9] Chen YJ, Wang PH, Yuan CC, Yen YK, Yang MJ, Ng HT, et al. Pregnancy following treatment of symptomatic myomas with laparoscopic bipolar coagulation of uterine vessels. Hum Reprod 2003;18:1077–81.

[10] Holub Z, Mara M, Kuzel D, Jabor A, Maskova J, Eim J. Pregnancy outcomes after uterine artery occlusion: prospective multicentric study. Fertil Steril 2008;90:1886–91.

[11] Dubuisson JB, Fauconnier A, Fourchotte V, Babaki-Fard K, Coste J, Chapron C. Laparoscopic myomectomy: predicting the risk of conversion to an open procedure. Hum Reprod 2001;16:1726–31.

[12] Wang PH, Liu WM, Fuh JL, Chao HT, Chao KC, Yuan CC. Laparoscopic uterine vessel occlusion in the treatment of women with symptomatic uterine myomas with and without adding laparoscopic myomectomy: 4-year results. J Minim Invasive Gynecol 2008;15:712–8.

[13] Rock JA, Jones HW III. Te Linde's Operative Gynecology. 9th ed. Philadelphia: JB Lippincott, 2003:784.

[14] Oelsner G, Cohen SB, Soriano D, Admon D, Mashiach S, Carp H. Minimal surgery for the twisted ischaemic adnexa can preserve ovarian function. Hum Reprod 2003;18:2599–602.

[15] Wang CJ, Yuen LT, Han CM, Kay N, Lee CL, Soong YK. A transient occlusion uterine perfusion procedure to decrease operative blood loss in laparoscopic myomectomy. Chang Gung Med J 2008;31:463–8.

[16] Wang PH, Liu WM, Fuh JL, Chao HT, Yuan CC, Chao KC. Symptomatic myoma treated with laparoscopic uterine vessel occlusion and subsequent immediate myomectomy: which is the optimal surgical approach? Fertil Steril 2009;92:762–9.

[17] Liu WM, Wang PH, Chou CS, Tang WL, Want IT, Tzeng CR. Efficacy of combined laparoscopic uterine artery occlusion and myomectomy via minilaparotomy in the treatment of recurrent uterine myomas. Fertil Steril 2007;87:356–61.

[18] Fedele L, Parazzini F, Luchini L, Mezzopane R, Tozzi L, Villa L. Recurrence of myomas after myomectomy: a transvaginal ultrasonographic study. Hum Reprod 1995;10:1795–6.

[19] Rossetti A, Sizzi O, Soranna L, Cucinelli F, Mancuso S, Lanzone A. Long-term results of laparoscopic myomectomy: recurrence rate in comparison with abdominal myomectomy. Hum Reprod 2001;16:770–4.

[20] Yoo EH, Lee PI, Huh CY, Kim DH, Lee BS, Lee JK, et al. Predictors of leiomyoma recurrence after laparoscopic myomectomy. J Minim Invasive Gynecol 2007;14:690–7.

[21] Lee CH, Chang CC, Kuo YT. Color Doppler evaluation of blood flow changes in leiomyomas after uterine artery ligation. Int J Gynaecol Obstet 2005;90:118–22.

[22] Lin WM. Laparoscopic bipolar coagulation of uterine vessels to treat symptomatic leiomyomas. J Am Assoc Gynecol Laparosc 2000;7:125–9.

[23] Park KH, Kim JY, Shin JS, Kwon JY, Koo JS, Jeong KA, et al. Treatment outcomes of uterine artery embolization and laparoscopic uterine artery ligation for uterine myoma. Yonsei Med J 2003;44: 694–702.

[24] Tulandi T, Murray C, Guralnick M. Adhesion formation and reproductive outcome after myomectomy and second-look laparoscopy. Obstet Gynecol 1993;82:213–5.

[25] Hanly EJ, Mendoza-Sagaon M, Murata K, Hardacre JM, De Maio A, Talamini MA. CO_2 pneumoperitoneum modifies the inflammatory response to sepsis. Ann Surg 2003;237:343–50.

[26] Seinera P, Arisio R, Decko A, Farina C, Crana F. Laparoscopic myomectomy: indications, surgical technique and complications. Hum Reprod 1997;12:1927–30.

[27] Dowson HM, Bong JJ, Lovell DP, Worthington TR, Karanjia ND, Rockall TA. Reduced adhesion formation following laparoscopic versus open colorectal surgery. Br J Surg 2008;95:909–14.

[28] Sileri P, Sthory R, McVeigh E, Child T, Cunningham C, Mortensen NJ, et al. Adhesions are common and costly after open pouch surgery. J Gastrointest Surg 2008;12:1039–45.

[29] Baakdah H, Tulandi T. Adhesions in gynecology complication, cost, and prevention: a review. Surg Technol Int 2005;14:185–90.

Chapter 3

Uterine Artery Embolization as an Alternative to Hysterectomy, in Patients with Uterine Myomas

Georgios Androutsopoulos, Dimitris Karnabatidis,
Georgios Michail and Georgios Decavalas

Additional information is available at the end of the chapter

http://dx.doi.org/10.5772/60845

Abstract

Uterine artery embolization (UAE) is a minimal invasive technique that uses transcutaneous common femoral artery approach to block uterine blood supply.

The aim of the procedure is to occlude or markedly reduce blood flow in both uterine arteries at the arteriolar level. This causes irreversible ischemia and leads to necrosis and subsequent shrinkage of uterine myomas.

In current clinical practice, uterine artery embolization represents an acceptable alternative to hysterectomy and myomectomy.

Keywords: Uterine artery embolization, selection criteria, effectiveness, complications

1. Introduction

Uterine artery embolization (UAE) is a minimal invasive technique that uses transcutaneous common femoral artery approach to block uterine blood supply.[1] It is based on established techniques for treating pelvic bleeding.[2]

It was first described in 1976, for the treatment of abnormal uterine bleeding in patients with gynecological malignancies.[3] Several years later, in 1994, UAE has been used preoperatively in patients with uterine myomas in order to reduce intraoperative blood loss and decrease transfusion requirements.[1, 4, 5] One year later, in 1995, UAE was introduced in patients with uterine myomas as an alternative approach to avoid surgical operation.[1, 4]

INTECH
open science | open minds

© 2015 The Author(s). Licensee InTech. This chapter is distributed under the terms of the Creative Commons Attribution License (http://creativecommons.org/licenses/by/3.0), which permits unrestricted use, distribution, and reproduction in any medium, provided the original work is properly cited.

In recent years, UAE represents an acceptable alternative to hysterectomy and myomectomy. [2, 6-8]

2. Technique

The procedure is usually performed under intravenous conscious sedation. Using the transcutaneous unilateral common femoral artery approach where both uterine arteries are selectively catheterized with a catheter or micro-catheter.[1, 4]

Following the sterile preparation of the right groin and local anesthesia, an arterial sheath (4–6 French) is introduced in the right common femoral artery using the Seldinger technique.[4] An angiography is then performed, in order to manipulate a visceral angiography catheter into the left internal iliac artery [Figure 1].[4]

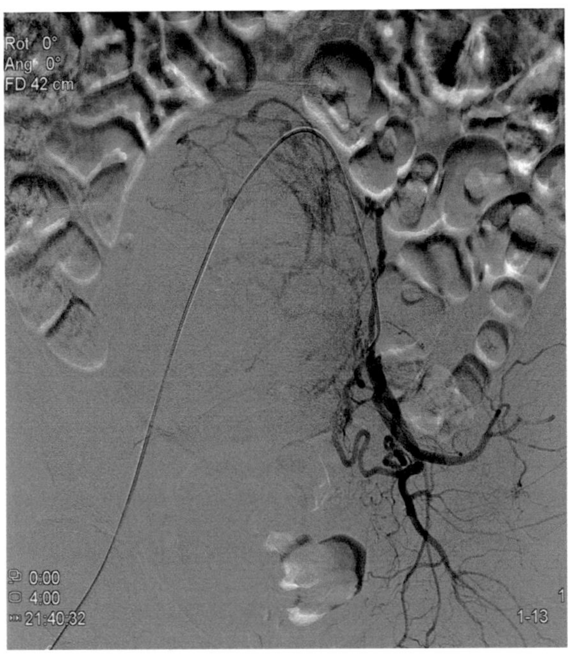

Figure 1. After insertion of the sheath, an angiography is performed to manipulate a visceral angiography catheter into the contralateral internal iliac artery.

Thereafter, a new angiography is performed in the contralateral oblique projection in order to identify the origin of the left uterine artery.[4] Then, the angiography catheter, or a micro-catheter, is placed into the transverse segment of the left uterine artery [Figure 2].[4, 9] If it is technically feasible, the catheter tip should be placed beyond the origin of the cervicovaginal branch, excluding it from embolization.[4, 9]

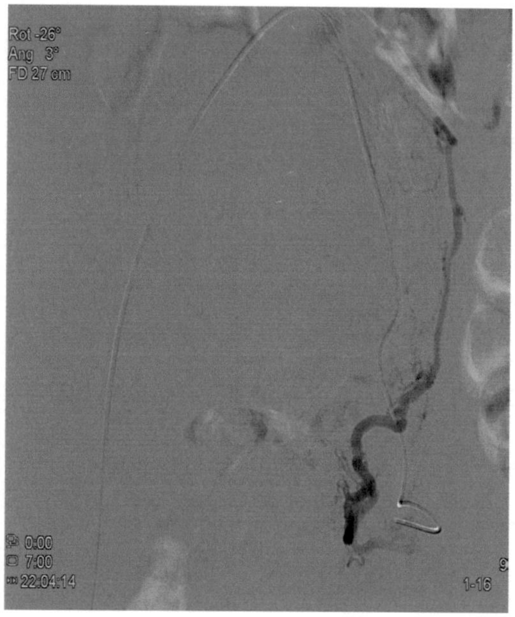

Figure 2. The angiography catheter or micro-catheter is illustrated, placed in the transverse segment of the uterine artery distal to the origin of cervicovaginal arteries.

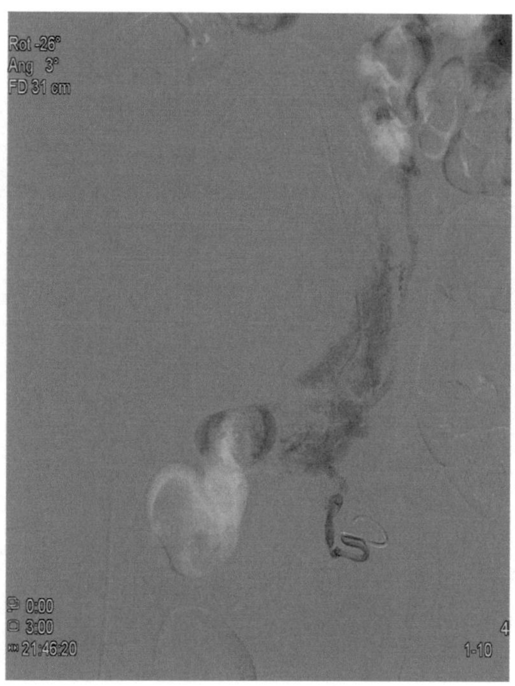

Figure 3. Following the correct positioning of the catheter or micro-catheter and under angiographic control, an embolic agent is then injected and UAE is performed.

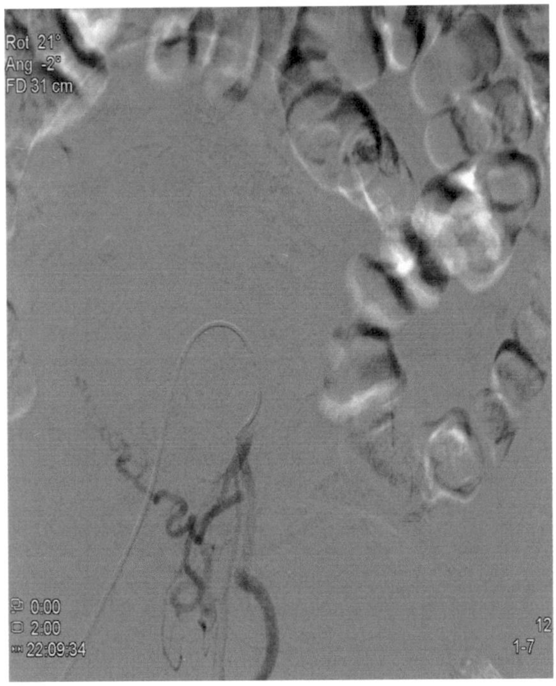

Figure 4. Subsequently the angiography catheter is manipulated into the ipsilateral internal iliac artery.

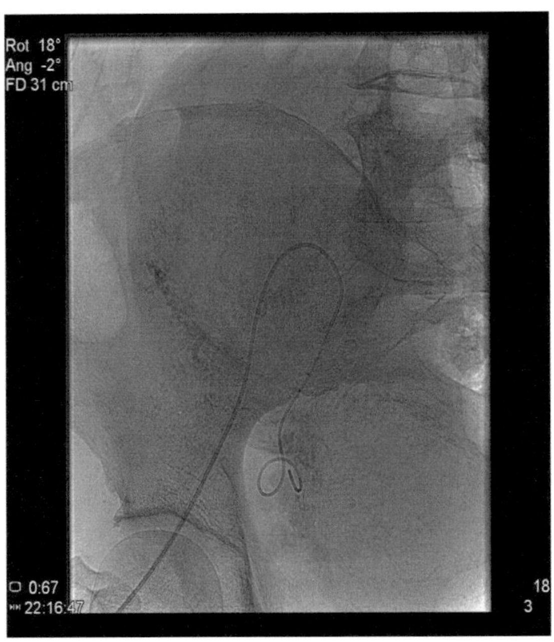

Figure 5. Finally the angiography catheter is placed in the lumen of the ipsilateral uterine artery.

http://dx.doi.org/10.5772/60845

Following the correct positioning of the catheter or micro-catheter and under angiographic control, an embolic agent (trisacryl gelatin microspheres, spherical polyvinyl alcohol) is injected and UAE is performed [Figure 3].[1, 2, 4, 9-11]

Subsequently, the angiography catheter is manipulated into the right internal iliac artery and placed in the right uterine artery [Figures 4, 5]. If this is not made possible, then the left common femoral artery is punctured and the procedure repeated.

Finally, when UAE has been completed, the catheter and sheath are removed. Hemostasis of the common femoral artery is achieved with manual compression.

The aim of UAE is to occlude or markedly reduce the blood flow in both uterine arteries at the arteriolar level.[2] This causes irreversible ischemia and leads to necrosis and the subsequent shrinkage of uterine myomas.[1, 2, 12]

3. Selection criteria

3.1. Indications

UAE is an alternative to hysterectomy in patients with uterine myomas.[2, 13] It is performed on appropriately selected patients who wish to preserve their uterus and avoid a surgical operation.[4, 6, 7, 10, 11, 13, 14]

A point of special interest is that UAE can be performed in patients with relevant co-morbidities (obesity, coronary artery disease) and increased perioperative risk for hysterectomy.[2, 7, 8]

Moreover, it can be performed on patients who refuse blood transfusion (for health concerns or religious reasons).[13]

3.2. Contraindications

Conditions that represent absolute contraindications for an UAE procedure are: pregnancy, active pelvic inflammatory disease, or other pelvic infection, genital cancer, history of pelvic radiation and impaired immune status [Table 1].[2, 4, 6, 10, 11, 14, 15]

Absolute contraindications	Relative contraindications
pregnancy	severe vascular disease limiting access
active pelvic inflammatory disease	severe allergy in radiographic contrast media
other pelvic infection	coagulopathy
genital cancer	impaired renal function
history of pelvic radiation	desire for future fertility
impaired immune status	

Table 1. Contraindications for uterine artery embolization.[2, 4, 6, 10, 11, 14-16]

Relative contraindications for UAE procedure are: severe vascular disease limiting access and catheter manipulations, severe allergy in radiographic contrast media, coagulopathy, impaired renal function, and desire for future fertility [Table 1].[2, 4, 6, 10, 11, 14-16]

The size and location of uterine myomas should also be considered in the patient selection process.[2]

4. Treatment advantages

UAE is a safe and effective technique for appropriately selected patients.[4, 6, 10, 14] It is a percutaneous procedure that involves no general anesthesia and no surgical incisions.[13]

The mean operative time is significantly shorter for patients treated with UAE than for hysterectomy patients (79 minutes vs. 95.4 minutes).[17, 18]

Intraprocedural blood loss is significantly less among patients treated with UAE, than among hysterectomy patients (30.9 ml vs 436.1 ml).[17, 18] As a result, blood transfusion requirements are significantly lower for patients treated with UAE than for hysterectomy patients (0% vs. 10–13.3%).[17-19]

Postoperative pain score during the first 24 hours is significantly less for patients treated with UAE than for hysterectomy patients.[17, 20, 21] However, postoperative pain during the entire hospital stay did not differ between the two groups (88.9% vs. 94.7%).[17, 18, 20, 21]

Febrile morbidity during hospital stay is significantly less common among patients treated with UAE than among hysterectomy patients (4.9% vs. 20%).[17, 18]

The length of hospital stay is significantly shorter for patients treated with UAE, than for hysterectomy patients (1–2 vs. 5–5.85 days).[13, 14, 17-19, 21] Recovery and return to normal activities are significantly swifter for patients treated with UAE than for hysterectomy patients (28.1 days vs. 63.4 days).[13, 14, 17-21]

The overall satisfaction rate among patients treated with UAE is high (80%–90%), comparing well with the satisfaction rate among hysterectomy patients.2 [13, 14, 17, 21, 22]

5. Treatment effectiveness

For the majority of patients treated with UAE, there is a substantial improvement in terms of symptoms and in quality of life aspects.[2, 4, 6, 10, 21] More specifically, there is reduction in bulk symptoms (88%–92%), elimination of abnormal uterine bleeding (>90%) and successful control of symptoms (75%).[2, 19]

Postoperatively among patients treated with UAE, there is a significant reduction in leiomyoma (50%–60%) and uterine (40%–50%) volumes.[2, 13, 19, 23] In the majority of cases, the reduction in leiomyoma and uterine volumes becomes noticeable in several weeks and sustains for 3–12 months after UAE.[2, 13, 23]

The effect of UAE on ovarian reserve is not well-established.[24] Follicle stimulating hormone (FSH) levels have no significant differences between patients treated with UAE and hysterectomy patients.[24]

A forthcoming pregnancy is feasible in patients treated with UAE.[25, 26] However, close monitoring of the placental status is recommended.[25]

6. Postoperative complaints

Postoperative symptoms (bleeding, pain, and pressure complaints) during the first 6 weeks among patients treated with UAE are slightly more common than among hysterectomy patients.[17, 18, 20, 21]

The readmission rate during the first 6 weeks for patients treated with UAE, is 11.1%; significantly higher than what it is for hysterectomy patients.[17, 18] However, since most readmissions in patients treated with UAE occurred at a time when patients treated with hysterectomy had not been yet discharged from the hospital, that figure might actually represent an overestimation.[18]

Readmissions for patients treated with UAE are mostly for: pain (22.2%), febrile morbidity (22.2%), or a combination of both (44.4%).[17, 18] Most of them occurred within the first week after discharge (77.8%), underlining the need for adequate postoperative follow-up during this period.[18]

Unscheduled hospital visits during the first 6 weeks are more common among patients treated with UAE than in patients treated with hysterectomy (32.5%–37% vs. 20%–25.3%).[17-19]

7. Treatment failure

The secondary intervention rate at 2 years of follow up is significantly higher among patients treated with UAE than among hysterectomy patients (23.5% vs. 8.0%).[17, 21, 23]

The secondary intervention rate at 5 years of follow up is significantly higher among patients treated with UAE than among hysterectomy patients (28.4% vs. 10.7%).[17, 21, 22]

Most of the secondary interventions on patients treated with UAE (77.2%) occur during the first 2 years of follow up.[14, 17, 22, 23]

There are many possible reasons for a UAE failure.[13, 27] Perhaps an incomplete uterine artery infarction results in regrowth of uterine myomas despite an initial reduction.[13, 27] Otherwise, UAE preserves apparently normal myometrium that may give rise to new uterine myomas.[13]

8. Complications

8.1. Intraprocedural complications

Overall, the intraprocedural complication rate does not differ significantly between patients treated with UAE and hysterectomy patients (8.6%–25% vs. 2.7%–20%).[17-19]

	Intraprocedural complications	Early postprocedural complications	Late postprocedural complications
Major complications	pulmonary embolism	pneumonia	
		sepsis	
		deep venous thrombosis	
		fibroid expulsion (requiring reintervention)	
		death	
		uterine necrosis	
		non-target embolization	
		vesicouterine fistula	
		small bowel volvulus	
		acute renal failure	
Minor complications	arterial spasm	vaginal discharge	permanent amenorrhea
	postpuncture hematoma	pain/fever (requiring readmission)	transient amenorrhea
	nerve injury at puncture site	fibroid expulsion (not requiring intervention)	prolonged vaginal discharge
	allergy in radiographic contrast media	postpuncture hematoma	
	nephrotoxicity	urinary tract infection	
	uterine artery dissection during catheterization	urinary retention	
	gluteal artery perforation	renoureteral colic	
	formation of blood clot in the gluteal artery	urinary incontinence	
		endometritis	
		hot flashes	
		thigh paresthesia	

Table 2. Complications in patients treated with uterine artery embolization.[2, 11, 13, 18, 19]

The intraprocedural *minor* complication rate is significantly lower among patients treated with UAE than among hysterectomy patients (22.2% vs. 30.7%).[18] The most common intraprocedural *minor* complications in patients treated with UAE are: arterial spasm, postpuncture hematoma, nerve injury at the puncture site, allergy in the radiographic contrast media, nephrotoxicity, and uterine artery dissection during catheterization [Table 2].[2, 11, 13, 18, 19] Other rare intraprocedural *minor* complications are: gluteal artery perforation and formation of blood clot in the gluteal artery [Table 2].[2, 11, 13, 18, 19]

The intraprocedural *major* complication rate has no significant differences between patients treated with UAE and hysterectomy patients (1.2% vs 1.3%).[18] Pulmonary embolism represents the most common intraprocedural *major* complication for patients treated with UAE [Table 2].[18]

8.2. Early postprocedural complications (up to 6 weeks)

Overall, the early postprocedural complication rate is significantly higher among patients treated with UAE than among hysterectomy patients (72% vs. 45%).[19]

The early postprocedural *minor* complication rate is significantly higher among patients treated with UAE, than among hysterectomy patients (58% vs. 40%).[18] The most common early postprocedural *minor* complications among patients treated with UAE are: vaginal discharge, pain/fever (requiring readmission), fibroid expulsion (not requiring intervention), postpuncture hematoma, urinary tract infection, urinary retention, renoureteral colic, urinary incontinence, endometritis, hot flashes, and thigh paresthesia [Table 2].[2, 11, 13, 18, 19]

The early postprocedural *major* complication rate is also higher among patients treated with UAE than among hysterectomy patients (3.7% vs. 1,3%).[18] The most common early postprocedural *major* complications among patients treated with UAE are: pneumonia, sepsis, deep venous thrombosis, and fibroid expulsion (requiring reintervention) [Table 2].[11, 18, 19] Other rare early postprocedural *major* complications are: death (secondary to septic shock, pulmonary embolism, non-target embolization), uterine necrosis, non-target inadvertent embolization (buttock necrosis, labial necrosis), vesicouterine fistula, small bowel volvulus, and acute renal failure [Table 2].[2, 13, 28]

8.3. Late postprocedural complications (up to 6 months)

The most common late postprocedural minor complications after UAE are: permanent amenorrhea (3.9%) and prolonged vaginal discharge (2%–17%) [Table 2].[2, 11, 13, 18, 28]

Transient amenorrhea after UAE is usually limited to a few cycles and it is not considered as a genuine complication.[2] Permanent amenorrhea after UAE occurs much more frequently in patients older than 45 years.[2, 13]

9. Postembolization syndrome

The syndrome is characterized by the occurrence of: pelvic pain, low-range pyrexia, nausea, vomiting, loss of appetite, and malaise.[2, 13] It primarily occurs the first few days after the procedure.[2, 13] It has a variable degree of intensity.[2]

It probably results from the release of cytokines related to ischemia and necrosis of uterine myomas.[2]

The postembolization syndrome is not considered as a complication of the UAE procedure.[2] However, in many cases it can result in prolonged hospitalization (beyond 48 hours), readmissions, and unexpected increase in the required level of care.[11]

10. Pregnancy after UAE

Full-term pregnancy is feasible for patients treated with UAE.[25, 26] However, there is increased risk of obstetric complications (miscarriage, abnormal placentation, preterm labor, malpresentation, and postpartum hemorrhage) for patients treated with UAE.[13, 25, 26, 29]

In particular, close monitoring of placental status is recommended for pregnant patients following UAE.[25, 26]

11. Conclusion

It is obvious that nonsurgical management of uterine myomas has shown promising results, simplifying or eliminating the need for surgical intervention in carefully selected patients.[7] However, it is not the treatment of choice for infertile women and for women wanting to preserve future childbearing capability. [7, 8 30]

Author details

Georgios Androutsopoulos[1*], Dimitris Karnabatidis[2], Georgios Michail[1] and Georgios Decavalas[1]

*Address all correspondence to: androutsopoulosgeorgios@hotmail.com

1 Department of Obstetrics and Gynaecology, University of Patras, Medical School, Rion, Greece

2 Department of Interventional Radiology, University of Patras, Medical School, Rion, Greece

We declare that we have no conflict of interest.

References

[1] Ravina J, Herbreteau D, Ciraru-Vigneron N, Bouret J, Houdart E, Aymard A, et al. Arterial embolisation to treat uterine myomata. Lancet 1995;346(8976):671–2.

[2] Stokes L, Wallace M, Godwin R, Kundu S, Cardella J. Quality improvement guidelines for uterine artery embolization for symptomatic leiomyomas. J Vasc Interv Radiol 2010;21(8):1153–63.

[3] Brault B, Marsault C, Moulin JD, Salmon R, Merland JJ. [Arterial embolization in the treatment of metrorrhagia of tumoral origin]. La Nouvelle presse medicale 1976;5(16):1043–6.

[4] Gonsalves C. Uterine artery embolization for treatment of symptomatic fibroids. Semin Intervent Radiol 2008;25(4):369–77.

[5] Ravina J, Merland J, Herbreteau D, Houdart E, Bouret J, Madelenat P. Preoperative embolization of uterine fibroma. Preliminary results (10 cases). Presse Med 1994;23(33):1540.

[6] Goodwin S, Spies J, Worthington-Kirsch R, Peterson E, Pron G, Li S, et al. Uterine artery embolization for treatment of leiomyomata: long-term outcomes from the FIBROID Registry. Obstet Gynecol 2008;111(1):22–33.

[7] Androutsopoulos G. How effective are current treatment strategies, in patients with uterine myomas? J Community Med Health Edu 2012;2(6):e107.

[8] Androutsopoulos G, Decavalas G. Management of uterine myomas: a critical update. Int J Transl Commun Med 2014;2:501.

[9] Worthington-Kirsch R. Uterine artery embolization: state of the art. Semin Intervent Radiol 2004;21(1):37–42.

[10] ACOG. ACOG practice bulletin. Alternatives to hysterectomy in the management of leiomyomas. Obstet Gynecol 2008;112(2 Pt 1):387–400.

[11] Goodwin S, Bonilla S, Sacks D, Reed R, Spies J, Landow W, et al. Reporting standards for uterine artery embolization for the treatment of uterine leiomyomata. J Vasc Interv Radiol 2003;14(9 Pt 2):S467–76.

[12] Colgan T, Pron G, Mocarski E, Bennett J, Asch M, Common A. Pathologic features of uteri and leiomyomas following uterine artery embolization for leiomyomas. Am J Surg Pathol 2003;27(2):167–77.

[13] Bradley L. Uterine fibroid embolization: a viable alternative to hysterectomy. Am J Obstet Gynecol 2009;201(2):127–35.

[14] Gupta J, Sinha A, Lumsden M, Hickey M. Uterine artery embolization for symptomatic uterine fibroids. Cochrane Database Syst Rev 2006;25(1):CD005073.

[15] SOGC. SOGC clinical practice guidelines. Uterine fibroid embolization (UFE). Number 150. Int J Gynaecol Obstet 2005;89(3):305–18.

[16] Usadi R, Marshburn P. The impact of uterine artery embolization on fertility and pregnancy outcome. Curr Opin Obstet Gynecol 2007;19(3):279–83.

[17] van der Kooij S, Bipat S, Hehenkamp W, Ankum W, Reekers J. Uterine artery embolization versus surgery in the treatment of symptomatic fibroids: a systematic review and metaanalysis. Am J Obstet Gynecol 2011;205(4):317.e1–18.

[18] Hehenkamp W, Volkers N, Donderwinkel P, de Blok S, Birnie E, Ankum W, et al. Uterine artery embolization versus hysterectomy in the treatment of symptomatic uterine fibroids (EMMY trial): Peri- and postprocedural results from a randomized controlled trial. Am J Obstet Gynecol 2005;193(5):1618–29.

[19] Pinto I, Chimeno P, Romo A, Paul L, Haya J, de la Cal M, et al. Uterine fibroids: uterine artery embolization versus abdominal hysterectomy for treatment—a prospective, randomized, and controlled clinical trial. Radiology 2003;226(2):425–31.

[20] Hehenkamp W, Volkers N, Birnie E, Reekers J, Ankum W. Pain and return to daily activities after uterine artery embolization and hysterectomy in the treatment of symptomatic uterine fibroids: Results from the randomized EMMY trial. Cardiovasc Intervent Radiol 2006;29(2):179–87.

[21] Edwards R, Moss J, Lumsden M, Wu O, Murray L, Twaddle S, et al. Uterine-artery embolization versus surgery for symptomatic uterine fibroids. N Engl J Med 2007;356(4):360–70.

[22] van der Kooij S, Hehenkamp W, Volkers N, Birnie E, Ankum W, Reekers J. Uterine artery embolization vs hysterectomy in the treatment of symptomatic uterine fibroids: 5-year outcome from the randomized EMMY trial. Am J Obstet Gynecol 2010;203(2):105.e1–13.

[23] Volkers N, Hehenkamp W, Birnie E, Ankum W, Reekers J. Uterine artery embolization versus hysterectomy in the treatment of symptomatic uterine fibroids: 2 years' outcome from the randomized EMMY trial. Am J Obstet Gynecol 2007;196(6):519.e1–11.

[24] van der Kooij S, Ankum W, Hehenkamp W. Review of nonsurgical/minimally invasive treatments for uterine fibroids. Curr Opin Obstet Gynecol 2012;24(6):368–75.

[25] Pron G, Mocarski E, Bennett J, Vilos G, Common A, Vanderburgh L. Pregnancy after uterine artery embolization for leiomyomata: The Ontario multicenter trial. Obstet Gynecol 2005;105(1):67–76.

[26] Walker W, McDowell S. Pregnancy after uterine artery embolization for leiomyomata: A series of 56 completed pregnancies. Am J Obstet Gynecol 2006;195(5):1266–71.

[27] Kroencke T, Scheurig C, Poellinger A, Gronewold M, Hamm B. Uterine artery embolization for leiomyomas: Percentage of infarction predicts clinical outcome. Radiology 2010;255(3):834–41.

[28] Toor S, Jaberi A, Macdonald D, McInnes M, Schweitzer M, Rasuli P. Complication rates and effectiveness of uterine artery embolization in the treatment of symptomatic leiomyomas: a systematic review and meta-analysis. AJR Am J Roentgenol 2012;199(5):1153-63.

[29] Goldberg J, Pereira L, Berghella V, Diamond J, Darai E, Seinera P, et al. Pregnancy outcomes after treatment for fibromyomata: uterine artery embolization versus laparoscopic myomectomy. Am J Obstet Gynecol 2004;191(1):18-21.

[30] Olive D, Lindheim S, Pritts E. Non-surgical management of leiomyoma: impact on fertility. Curr Opin Obstet Gynecol 2004;16(3):239-43.

Chapter 4

Artery Embolization of Uterine Fibroids as Alternative to Hysterectomy

Chrisostomos Sofoudis

Additional information is available at the end of the chapter

http://dx.doi.org/10.5772/60473

Abstract

Uterine artery embolization (UAE) was presented as a treatment for symptomatic uterine fibroids in the early of 1990s, after initially being used as a temporary surgical procedure before the performance of hysterectomy or myomectomy. Although the existence of intraoperative complications is associated with overall survival, plenty of these complications can be prevented. Until recently, surgical management represents the treatment of choice regarding the uterine fibroids. With the arrival of UAE, the percentage of major complications such as intraoperative bleeding, adhesions and ureteral injury is decreasing. The ultimate scope of the problem remains the proper management accompanied by knowledge and experience.

Keywords: Uterine embolization, fibroids, hysterectomy

1. Introduction

1.1. Uterine fibroids

Uterine fibroids are very common, non-cancerous (benign) growths that develop in the muscular wall of the uterus. Other names for fibroids include Leiomyoma, Leiomyomata, Fibromyomas, Fibromas, Myofibromas, and Myomas. They are composed of smooth muscle and connective tissue developing and enhancing the uterus wall. They can present in a very wide range of sizes, from small to enlarged myomas. Africans, in comparison with Caucasians, are three times more prone to uterine fibroids formation. They account for one third of all hysterectomies performed in the United States —approximately 100,000 procedures every

INTECH
open science | open minds

© 2015 The Author(s). Licensee InTech. This chapter is distributed under the terms of the Creative Commons Attribution License (http://creativecommons.org/licenses/by/3.0), which permits unrestricted use, distribution, and reproduction in any medium, provided the original work is properly cited.

year. Due to their enlarged size, fibroids deform the abdominal cavity. In most cases, more than one are detected inside the peritoneal wall.

Due to their location, uterine fibroids can be classified into the following categories:

a. **Submucosal fibroids.** Fibroids that grow into the inner cavity of the uterus (submucosal fibroids) are more likely to cause prolonged, heavy menstrual bleeding and infertility problems for women trying to achieve a pregnancy.

b. **Subserosal fibroids.** Fibroids that project to the outside of the uterus (subserosal fibroids) can sometimes press on the bladder, causing urinary symptoms. If fibroids bulge from the back of the uterus, they occasionally can press into either the rectum, causing a pressure sensation, or the spinal nerves, causing backache.

c. **Intramural fibroids.** Some fibroids grow within the muscular uterine wall (intramural fibroids). If they are large enough, they can distort the shape of the uterus and cause prolonged, heavy menstrual cycles, as well as pain and pressure.

According to the size, the symptomatology can vary from pressure to abdominal pain and signs of peritoneal obstruction. Vaginal bleeding accompanied with episodes of metrorrhagia, especially in premenopausal women could disturb their daily activities and their quality of life. Other symptoms comprise heavy, prolonged menstrual periods and unusual monthly bleeding, sometimes with clots; this medical situation could lead to anaemia. Fibroids' existence may also be detected via pain in the back and legs, pain during sexual intercourse, bladder pressure leading to a frequent urge to urinate, and pressure on the bowel, leading to constipation and bloating.

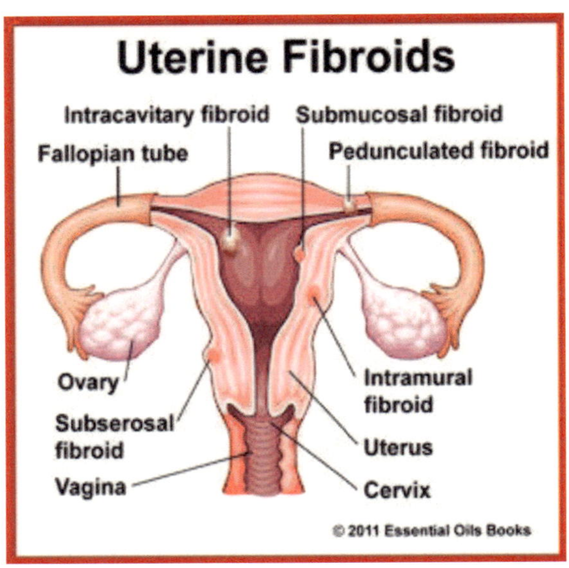

Figure 1. Classification of uterine fibroids (2011 Essential Oils Books.)

2. Diagnostic procedures

The diagnosis of uterine fibroids could be made via the taking of a detailed medical history, an assiduous physical examination, and proper imaging techniques. The anamnesis history may also include details such as the age of the patient, possible anomalies of the menstrual cycle, episodes of abdominal pain, and urgent pressure resulting from incontinence. Information on factors such as episodes of metrorraghia and diffuse vaginal bleeding could produce a successful diagnosis. The role of transvaginal ultrasonography in diagnosis is unquestionable.

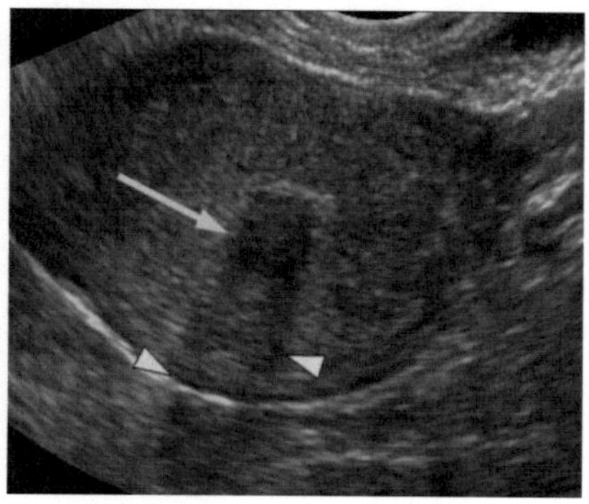

Figure 2. Ultrasonographic depiction of uterine fibroid.(Arrow). Wilde Sue and Scott-Barrett Sarah. Radiological appearances of uterine fibroids. Indian J Radiol Imaging. Aug 2009; 19(3): 222–231.

Uterine fibroids appear as well-defined solid masses with a similar echogenicity to the myometrium. They can deform the uterus' contour, resulting in a bulky formation. Submucous fibroids could be easily differentiated from the endometrium layer but not so easily from endometrial polyps. CT examination might not prefer to choose imaging regarding the diagnosis of pelvic masses. In many cases, uterine myomas reflect a bulky, deformed uterus or a mass in continuity with the uterus.

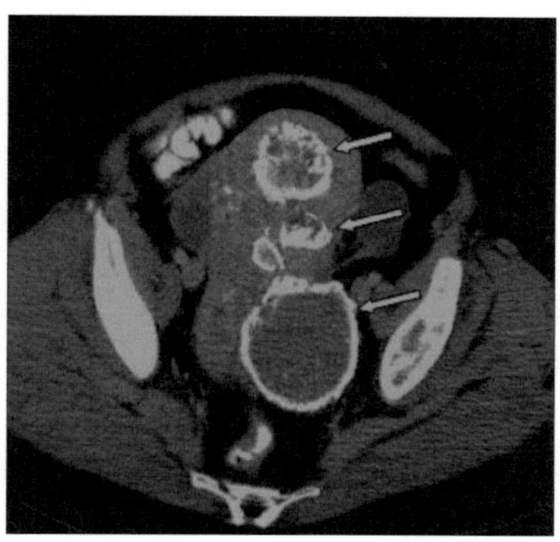

Figure 3. CT scan showing multiple uterine fibroids.(Arrows). Wilde Sue and Scott-Barrett Sarah. Radiological appearances of uterine fibroids. Indian J Radiol Imaging. Aug 2009; 19(3): 222–231.

The sensitivity and specificity of the MRI reflect on the accurate preoperative diagnosis of uterine myomas. The imaging findings consist of an excellent delineation of both internal and external uterine contours, measurement accuracy of intercornual diameter, visualization improvement of the endometrial architecture, and identification of uterine horns.

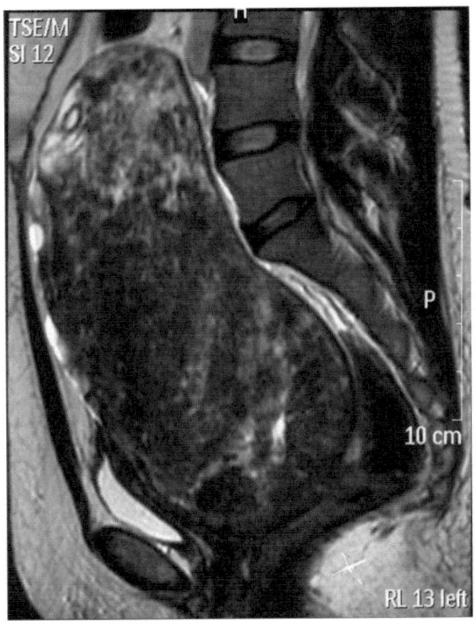

Figure 4. Sagittal T2 weighted MR image showing a large fibroid mass extending to upper endplate of lumbar spine. Madhuri TK, Kamran W,Walker W, Butler-Manuel S.Synchronous *uterine* artery embolization and laparoscopic myomectomy for massive *uterine* leiomyomas. JSLS.2010 Jan-Mar;14(1):120- 2.

3. Management options

Leiomyomas may develop in the myometrium cavity, occasionally in the cervix, broad ligament, and ovaries. Most frequently, they develop in the myometrial wall and could lead to uterine distortion. The treatment of choice consists of surgical or laparoscopical myomectomy avoiding all the intra- or postoperative complications. The advantages regarding laparoscopic myomectomy involve less blood loss, shorter hospital stays, and fewer intraoperative complications. The technical skill required for the excision of myoma and a lack of surgical experience are considered significant limiting factors to the wide acceptance of this technique.

Factors such as diffuse abdominal bleeding, adhesions, and multiple and enlarged myomas contraindicate the use of laparoscopic management. In cases of episodes of vaginal bleeding accompanied with abdominal pain, constipation, and ureter obstruction, the choice of a hysterectomy seems mandatory. Among all the intraoperative complications, the necessity of the treatment of the fibroid bleeding appears to be paramount. Specific research takes place continuously regarding the development of an ideal, minimally invasive method, trying to reach the goals of a treatment that is safe and tolerated well. Plenty of surgical or non-surgical methods have been performed, such as laparoscopic uterine ligation, myomectomy, and high-intensity, focused ultrasound. The arrival of uterine artery embolization (UAE) has changed all the therapeutical options. No limitations appear regarding the fibroids' size and number that can be treated with UAE.

4. Uterine arteries embolization

4.1. Basic principles

The embolization of uterine fibroids arteries represents a minimally invasive procedure as far as the treatment of uterine fibroids is concerned. Indications of uterine artery embolization are the following:

- Trauma
- Malignant gynaecological tumours
- Post-labour bleeding
- Bleeding following gynaecological surgery

This specific technique manages to be extended during the last two years enhancing the management of arterial venosus malformations of the genital tract and gestational trophoblastic disease. The limitations of uterine fibroid embolization (UFE) are many, and subsume women with no symptomatology regarding their condition, existence of cancer, or pelvic infection. Women with a known allergy to contrast materials should undergo preoperative treatment or follow a different treatment option. The gold standard is based on fibroid reduction by obstructing its vessels with embolic elements during the catheterization of uterine arteries. Through this procedure, a successful devascularization and prolonged quality of life can be achieved. The fibroid shrinkage may cause a significant decrease of all intra- or postoperative complications.

4.2. Equipment

Before the performance of the procedure, it is mandatory to perform a preoperative depiction of the uterine cavity, certifying that uterine fibroids are the main cause of the uterine bleeding, and the number, the size, and the location of uterine myomas. The appropriate information should consist of many details, such as gestational status, known allergies, reception of medications such as NSAIDs, and known medical status. The necessary equipment is the following:

- X-ray equipment
- Catheter

- Embolic material

The presence of fluoroscopy for the transformation of the X-rays into video depictions is obligatory. The catheter encloses a long plastic tube approximately 1/8 of the catheter in diameter. The necessary embolic agents are the following:

- Calibrated microspheres of 500, 700, and 900 μm, alone or in combination

- Gelfoam, a gelatine sponge material

All the mentioned substances certify the safety and effectiveness of the procedure regarding the uterine fibroid embolization. In conclusion, the necessity of an intravenous line and the monitoring of heartbeat and blood pressure should always be stressed. During the procedure, all the security instructions should be followed, achieving the prevention of all possible intraoperative complications.

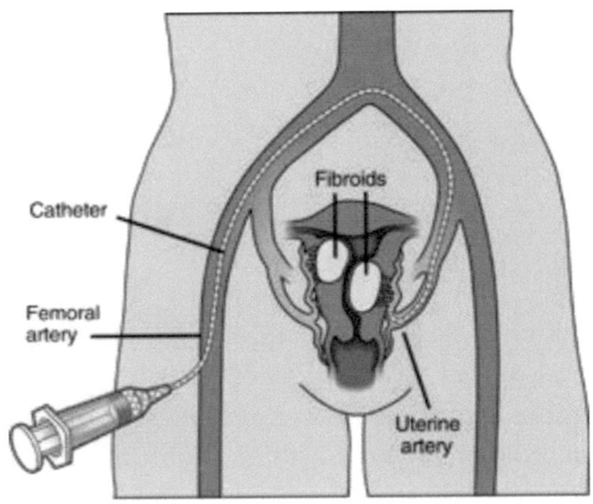

Figure 5. Procedure of uterine fibroid embolization (Medscape)

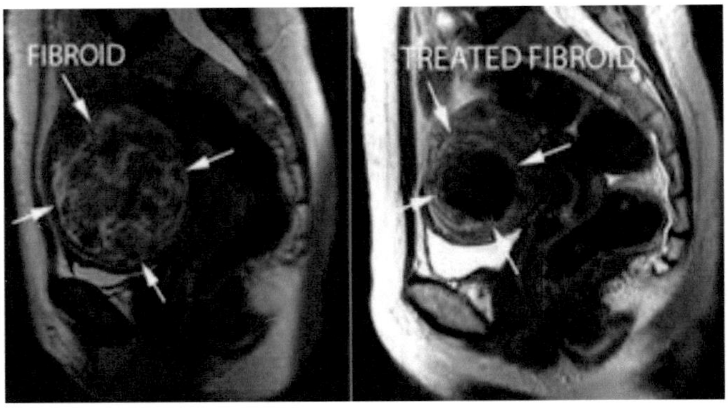

Figure 6. Left: A large fibroid is seen in the uterus (arrows). Right: Four months following uterine fibroid embolization, the fibroid has substantially decreased. (Fibroid.png)

http://dx.doi.org/10.5772/60473

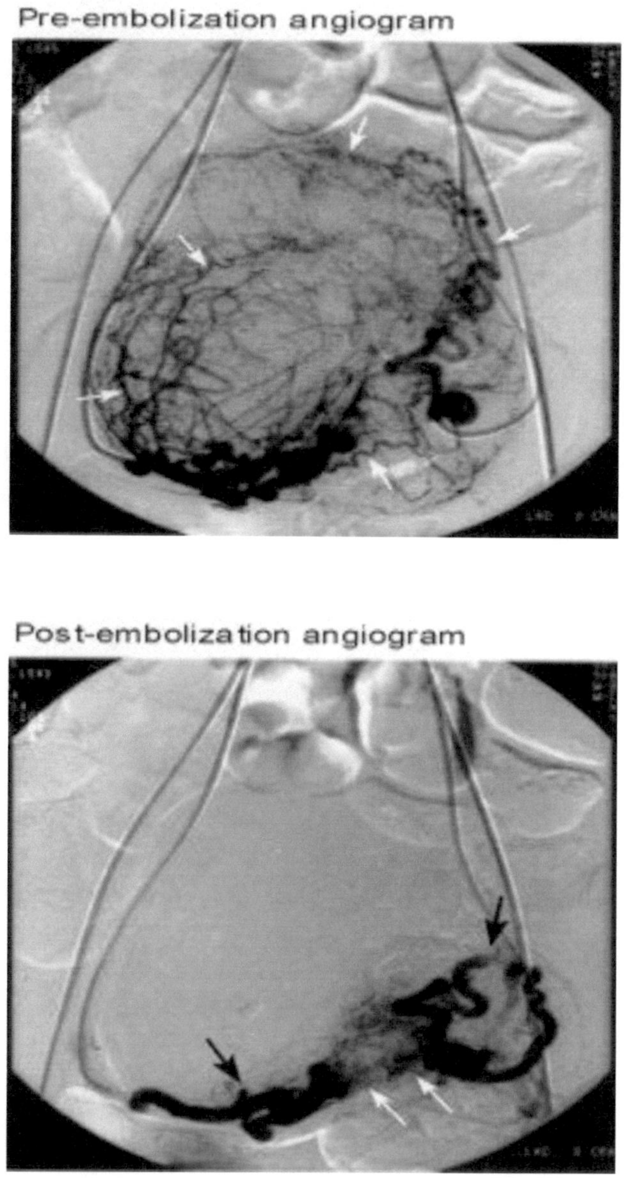

Figure 7. Uterine arteries embolization. Pre- and Post-embolization angiogram.(Georgetown University Hospital-Divison of Vascular and International Radiology)

4.3. Procedure

Transcatheter arterial embolization represents an alternative type of hysterectomy regarding the treatment of symptomatic uterine myomas. By the time the embolic agents are injected inside the uterine arteries, they can reach the entire arterial central branch, including the arterial in- and outflow. The successful collateral blood supply provides arterial flow, prohibiting the ischemic establishment of the area. The impact of the embolic agents could produce conditions of shrinkage throughout the uterine fibroids. This ischemic devascularization prohibits intraoperative bleeding and the following hysterectomy. The success rate depends on the skills and the expertise of the surgeon.

Additionally, blood pressure monitoring, oxygen flow, and available sedatives in case of pain during the injection appear necessary. The next step reflects the transformation of the X-ray guidance into video depiction. At the end of the procedure, the transarterial catheter is removed and a haemostasis of the area is achieved by applying local pressure. The majority of the women on whom this procedure was performed declared that they were satisfied: an average of 50%. The ultimate goal depends on the fertility rate regarding nulliparous premenopausal women. For women who are interested in future fertility, a myomectomy seem to be a suitable choice. In general, uterine fibroid embolization seems to be a safe procedure in correlation with all intraoperative instructions, minimizing all intra- or postoperative complications.

4.4. Complications

During the procedure of uterine arteries embolization concerning the treatment of uterine fibroids, many intra- or postoperative complications could emerge. The complication rate depends, as mentioned, on the skill and expertise of the surgeon. Infection, local bleeding, or local hematoma represent the earliest postoperative complications.

Allergic reactions or spasms of the uterine arteries with the after-effect of pain, due to contrast medium and local ischemia, can be treated with vasodilator agents or micro-catheter techniques. The intraoperative abdominal pain in terms of the local ischemia responds to NSAIDs. Postoperative infection followed in many cases, as local or diffuse sepsis caused by endometritis or tubo-ovarian abscess, which can be treated preoperatively with broad spectrum antibiotic agents according to established guidelines. In many cases, episodes of pain persistence over two weeks after the procedure have been reported. In these conditions, and in the case of an absence of infection, surgical intervention seems mandatory. The possibility of hysterectomy due to chronic abdominal pain is estimated in 2% of the women who underwent uterine embolization.

The procedure of uterine arteries embolization can lead to postembolization ovarian failure in women over 45. The pathophysiologic mechanisms remain unknown. The whole procedure is significant, mostly in cases of fertility preservation. The postoperative impact of uterine arteries embolization reflects the improvement of menstrual disorders. Improvement during episodes of menorrhagia and metrorrhagia has been reported. In many cases, the generated embolization can lead to amenorrhea due to ovarian failure. Uterine wall defects, episodes of uterine fistula or uterine necrosis represent neglected cases of uterine arteries embolization. Due to treatment failure, the possibility of hysterectomy performance after uterine arteries embolization appears as a reality. The main causes reflect the existence of persistent bleeding, abdominal pain, fibroid prolapse, and episodes of uterine malignancies.

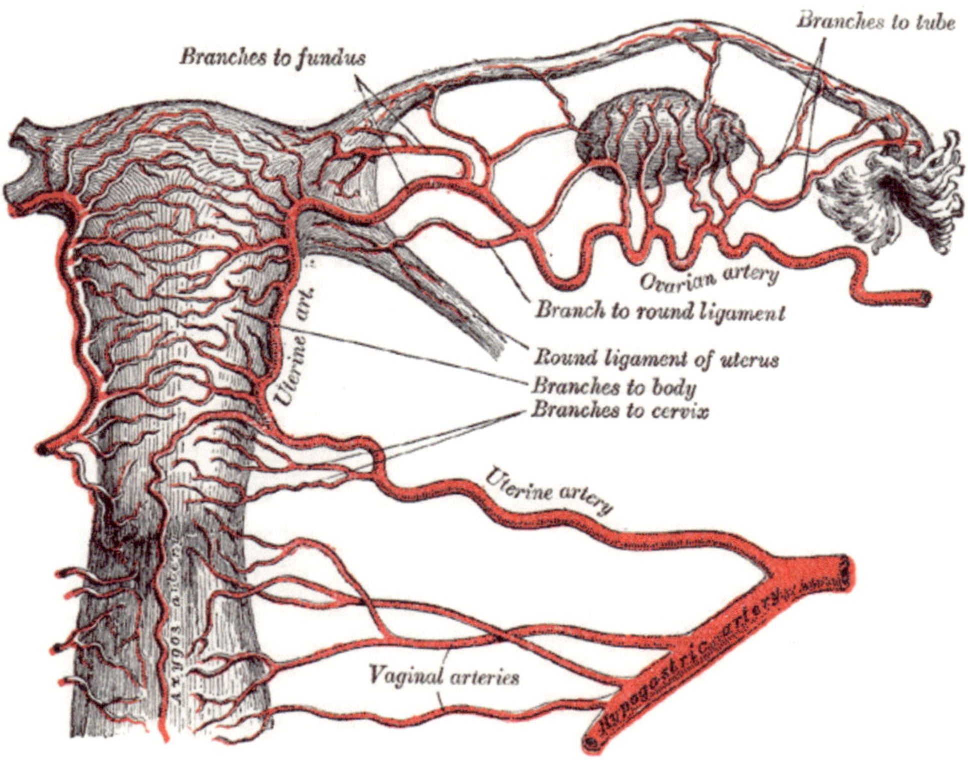

Figure 8. Arteries of the female reproductive tract (*posterior* view): *uterine artery*, *ovarian artery* and *vaginal arteries*. (Wikipedia)

4.5. Other techniques

The uterine arteries embolization regarding episodes of symptomatic uterine fibroids represents the treatment of choice in cases of diffuse intraoperative abdominal bleeding. Apart from this skilled and expertised procedure, alternative techniques such as ligation of uterine arteries or providing pharmaceutical agents such GnRH agonists with the ultimate scope being the increase of apoptosis among symptomatic fibroid muscle cells may emanate.

In cases of symptomatic uterine fibroids, focusing on fertility preservation via a laparoscopic ligation of uterine arteries seems to be a logical option. It reflects an effective procedure and stands as a worthy alternative to hysterectomy or myomectomy. Necessary conditions required for this procedure may be laparoscopic skills and the precise location of the uterine vessels. The collateral blood supply could lead to shrinkage due to ischaemia and infraction. The procedure can be performed laparoscopically or abdominally, though the laparoscopic procedure is superior. Every procedure has specific indications and contraindications. The crucial condition concerning the success rate increase remains the performance in centres with appropriate expertise in laparoscopic surgery. If these conditions cannot be fulfilled, massive abdominal bleeding could occur with the final result being the performance of a hysterectomy.

The existence of vaginal spotting after uterine ligation is considered to be a prohibitive factor. The second alternative procedure represents the supply of GnRH agonists with the principle example being the use of triptorelin. The pharmaceutical impact of GnRH agonists reflects the cell death, cell necrosis, and finally apoptosis. As result, all the apoptotic cells could lead to vessel obstruction and decrease of uterine flow. This procedure deputizes as its ultimate goal the fibroid shrinkage and the management of possible intraoperative bleeding. New strategies have been conducted in order to minimize the operative complications. The hysteroscopic endometrial ablation represents an alternative option. All these non-surgical procedures increase the fertility preservation in women of reproductive age.

Many studies must be further conducted, in order for precise and detailed results to emerge. The research steps must follow all the current guidelines focusing on the minimization of all intra- or postoperative complications. The ultimate goal remains the increase of survival rates and improvement of the surgical procedure. In comparison with all mentioned techniques, the B-Lynch technique represents an alternative procedure with remarkable results regarding fertility preservation and the management of operative bleeding after resection of uterine fibroids. The special advantage of this innovative technique is that it presents an alternative to major surgical procedures for controlling pelvic arterial pulse pressure, or hysterectomy. To date, this suturing technique, when applied correctly, has been successful with no problems and no apparent complications.

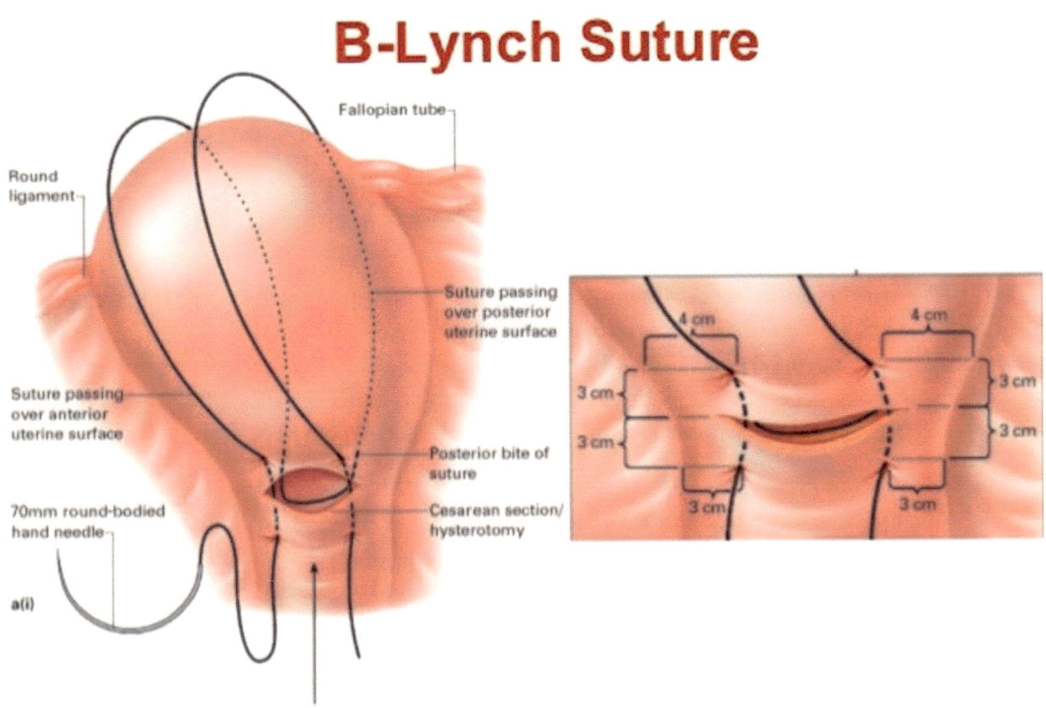

Figure 9. Schematic depiction of B-Lynch technique. (B-Lynch & Shah, A Comprehensive Text Book of PPH 2nd Ed. 2012)

5. Fertility preservation

The fibroid shrinkage due to uterine artery embolization in young nulliparous women, and especially the management of extensive metrorrhagia, involves important issues regarding fertility preservation. Due to the arrival of reports describing gestation and labour after uterine artery embolization (UAE), many alternative procedures have been performed.

Many studies reported individually with respect to postoperative complications. Many cases reported episodes of miscarriage, preterm deliveries, pre-eclampsia, and intrauterine growth restriction, as well a high incidence of caesarean sections. Finally, several cases of intrauterine adhesions, endometrial atrophy, and fistula creation between the uterine cavity and the embolized intramural myoma have been reported in the current literature. Despite all the intra- or postoperative complications, uterine artery embolization prevents hysterectomies. This procedure must be properly planned depending on the haemorrhagic conditions of the disease and the surgical expertise of the surgeon.

Uterine artery embolization (UAE) has gained a great impact due to its uterus preservation, a necessary condition regarding female psychological and reproductive status. Uterus preservation is related to female psychosocial integrity and decreases anxiety and depression in correlation with women who have undergone hysterectomies. Many studies have reported the correlation between the performance of hysterectomy, and psychological and bodily disorders. In our period, in a world characterized by anxiety, economical, and physical stress, and difficulties within human relationships, fertility preservation has a high value. Nulliparous women feel mutilated after the performance of a hysterectomy, unable to achieve the ultimate aim of childbirth. All these reports try to demystify concepts such as uterine artery embolization and fertility preservation. Multidisciplinary cooperation is mandatory for ultimate procedure management.

6. Patient counselling

The most significant factor for uterine artery embolization involves patient counselling. The patient must be informed regarding the procedure, all intra- or postoperative complications, as well as conditions which are related to fertility preservation and the increase of life expectancy. Prior to any management procedure, all patients need evaluation through their medical history and physical examination. Daily habits, reception of medicament agents, and menstrual disorders must be mentioned in order to make clear the correlation with the management options.

The next step will be the evaluation of the severity of the lesion. Imaging findings and laboratory examination could confirm the results from the physical examination. A basic principle will be the constant updating regarding all the predisposing factors, which could influence the management selection. The patient must understand all the possible management options, the mechanisms procedure, and decide on the ultimate management option.

The physician's duty will be analysis and understanding the condition's status. The final decision depends on the patient. A well-informed patient together with the medical stuff will map the proper procedure, taking into consideration not only the marital and reproductive status, but also the individual family planning of the patient.

All studies derived from the current bibliography agree that patient counselling could produce fewer intra- or postoperative complications and increase the life expectancy rate. Besides the preoperative patient counselling, an important role could be played by the well-trained psychologists and health professionals concerning the postoperative course. They should inform the patient regarding the postoperative options in order to prevent the possible stress and depression that could emerge. The postoperative mapping after uterine artery embolization as an alternative to a hysterectomy consists of future pregnancy. Many studies must be conducted in order to ensure future results.

7. Conclusion

Embolization of uterine arteries in cases of symptomatic fibroids introduces a vital and precise procedure in order to minimize all the intra- or postoperative complications, as well as to increase life expectancy and survival rates. Surgical skills, patient counselling, and properly trained medical staff should be taken into consideration as the proper indicators of the uterine arteries embolization. Multidisciplinary cooperation is mandatory with a view to proper and uneventful management.

Author details

Chrisostomos Sofoudis

Address all correspondence to: chrisostomos.sofoudis@gmail.com

2nd Department of Obstetrics and Gynaecology, University of Athens, Aretaieio Hospital, Greece

The author declares no financial interest regarding this manuscript.

References

[1] Chabbert-Buffet N, Esber N, Bouchard P. Fibroid growth and medical options for treatment. Fertil Steril. 2014 Sep; 102(3):630–9.

[2] Doherty L, Mutlu L, Sinclair D, Taylor H. Uterine fibroids: clinical manifestations and contemporary management. Reprod Sci. 2014 Sep; 21(9):1067–92.

[3] Bulun SE. Uterine fibroids. N Engl J Med. 2013 Oct 3; 369(14):1344–55.

[4] Lefebvre G, Vilos G, Allaire C, Jeffrey J. The management of uterine leiomyomas. SOgc clinical practice guideline, no.128, May 2003. J Obstet Gynecol Can 2003; 25(5): 396–405.

[5] Burbank F, Hutchings FL. Uterine artery occlusion by embolization or surgery for treatment of fibroids: a unifying hypothesis-transient uterine ischemia. J Am Assoc Gynecol Laparosc 2000; 7:S1–49.

[6] Walker WJ, Pelage JP. Uterine artery embolization for symptomatic fibroids: clinical results in 400 women with imaging follow-up.Br J Obstet Gynecol 2002; 109:1262–72.

[7] Spies JB, Spector A, Roth AR, Baker CM, Mauro L, Murphy-Skrynarz K. Complications after uterine artery embolization for leiomyomas. Obstet Gynecol 2002; 100(5): 873–80.

[8] Edwards RD, Moss JG, Lumdsen MA, et al. Uterine-artery embolization versus surgery for symptomatic uterine fibroids. N Engl J Med 2007; 356(4):360–70.

[9] Henenkamp WJ, Volkers NA, Birnie E, et al. Symptomatic uterine fibroids: treatment with uterine artery embolization or hysterectomy — results from the randomized clinical embolization versus hysterectomy (EMMY) Trial. Radiology. 2008; 246(3): 823–32.

[10] Pinto I, Chimeno P, Romo A, et al. Uterine fibroids: uterine artery embolization versus abdominal hysterectomy for treatment. A prospective, randomized and controlled clinical trial. Radiology.2003; 226(2):425–31.

[11] Wilde S, Scott S. Radiological appearances of uterine fibroids. Indian J Radiol Imaging. Aug 2009; 19(3): 222–231.

[12] Madhuri TK, Kamran W, Walker W, Butler-Manuel S.Synchronous uterine artery embolization and laparoscopic myomectomy for massive uterine leiomyomas. JSLS. 2010 Jan–Mar; 14(1):120–2.

[13] Pelage JP, Le Dref O, Soyer P, et al. Fibroid-related menorrhagia: treatment with superselective embolization of the uterine arteries and midterm follow-up. Radiology. 2000; 215(2):428–31.

[14] Pron G, Mocarski E, Cohen M, et al. Hysterectomy for complications after uterine artery embolization for leiomyoma: results of a Canadian multicenter clinical trial. J Am Assoc Gynecol Laparosc 2003; 10(1):99–106.

[15] Spies JB, Bradley LD, Guido R, Maxwell GL, Levine BA, Coyne K. Outcomes from leiomyoma therapies: comparison with normal controls. Obstet Gynecol 2010; 116(3): 641–652.

[16] Brunereau L, Herbreteau D, Gallas S, et al. Uterine artery embolization in the primary treatment of uterine leiomyomas: technical features and prospective follow-up with clinical and sonographic examinations in 58 patients. AJR Am J Roentgenol 2000; 175(5):1267–1272.

[17] Siskin GP, Shlansky-Goldberg RD, Goodwin SC, et al. UAE versus Myomectomy Study Group. A prospective multicenter comparative study between myomectomy and uterine artery embolization with polyvinyl alcohol microspheres: long-term clinical outcomes in patients with symptomatic uterine fibroids. J Vasc Interv Radiol 2006; 17(8):1287–1295.

[18] Ananthakrishnan G, Murray L, Ritchie M, et al. Randomized comparison of uterine artery embolization (UAE) with surgical treatment in patients with symptomatic uterine fibroids (REST trial): subanalysis of 5-year MRI findings. Cardiovasc Intervent Radiol 2013; 36(3):676–681.

[19] Ruuskanen A, Hippeläinen M, Sipola P, Manninen H. Uterine artery embolisation versus hysterectomy for leiomyomas: primary and 2-year follow-up results of a randomised prospective clinical trial. Eur Radiol 2010; 20(10):2524–2532.

[20] Jun F, Yamin L, Xinli X, et al. Uterine artery embolization versus surgery for symptomatic uterine fibroids: a randomized controlled trial and a meta-analysis of the literature. Arch Gynecol Obstet 2012; 285(5):1407–1413.

[21] van der Kooij SM, Bipat S, Hehenkamp WJ, Ankum WM, Reekers JA. Uterine artery embolization versus surgery in the treatment of symptomatic fibroids: a systematic review and metaanalysis. Am J Obstet Gynecol 2011; 205(4):e1–e18.

[22] Gupta JK, Sinha A, Lumsden MA, Hickey M. Uterine artery embolization for symptomatic uterine fibroids. Cochrane Database Syst Rev 2012; 5:CD005073.

[23] Poulsen B, Munk T, Ravn P. Long-term follow up after uterine artery embolization for symptomatic uterine leiomyomas. Acta Obstet Gynecol Scand 2011; 90(11):1281–1283.

[24] Popovic M, Berzaczy D, Puchner S, Zadina A, Lammer J, Bucek RA. Long-term quality of life assessment among patients undergoing uterine fibroid embolization. AJR Am J Roentgenol 2009; 193(1):267–27.

[25] Cardozo ER, Clark AD, Banks NK, Henne MB, Stegmann BJ, Segars JH. The estimated annual cost of uterine leiomyomata in the United States. Am J Obstet Gynecol. 2012; 206(3):211–e1–9.

[26] Yoon SW, Kim KA, Cha SH, Kim YM, Lee C, Na YJ, et al. Successful use of magnetic resonance-guided focused ultrasound surgery to relieve symptoms in a patient with symptomatic focal adenomyosis. Fertil Steril. 2008; 90(5):2018. e13–5.

[27] Behera MA, Leong M, Johnson L, Brown H. Eligibility and accessibility of magnetic resonance-guided focused ultrasound (MRgFUS) for the treatment of uterine leiomyomas. Fertil Steril. 2010; 94(5):1864–8.

[28] O'Sullivan AK, Thompson D, Chu P, Lee DW, Stewart EA, Weinstein MC. Cost-effectiveness of magnetic resonance guided focused ultrasound for the treatment of uterine fibroids. Int J Technol Assess Health Care. 2009; 25(1):14–25.

[29] Zowall H, Cairns JA, Brewer C, Lamping DL, Gedroyc WM, Regan L. Cost-effectiveness of magnetic resonance-guided focused ultrasound surgery for treatment of uterine fibroids. Bjog. 2008; 115(5):653–62.

[30] Tropeano G, Amoroso S, Scambia G. Non-surgical management of uterine fibroids. Hum Reprod Update. 2008; 14(3):259–74.

[31] Hald K, Langebrekke A, Klow NE, Noreng HJ, Berge AB, Istre O. Laparoscopic occlusion of uterine vessels for the treatment of symptomatic fibroids: initial experience and comparison to uterine artery embolization. Am J Obstet Gynecol. 2004; 190: 37–43.

[32] Watkinson A, Nicholson A. Uterine artery embolization to treat symptomatic uterine fibroids. BMJ. 2007; 335(7622):720–722.

[33] Marshburn PB, Matthews ML, Hurst BS. Uterine artery embolization as a treatment option for uterine myomas. Obstet Gynecol Clin North Am.2006; 33(1):125–144.

[34] Smith WJ, Upton E, Shuster EJ, Klein AJ, Schawrz ML. Patient satisfactory and disease specific quality of life after uterine artery embolization Am J Obstet Gynecol 2004; 190(6):1697–1703.

[35] Pritts EA. Fibroids and infertility: a systematic review of the evidence. Obstetricial and Gynecological Survey, 2001, vol.56, no.8, pp. 483-491.

[36] Poncelet C, Benifla JL, Batallan A, Darai E, Mandelenat P. Myoma and infertility :analysis of the literature. Gynecol Obset Fertil, 2001, vol.29, no.6, pp. 413–421.

[37] Fletcher H, Wharfe G, Williams N, Gordon-strachan G, Pedican M, Brooks A. Venous thromboembolism as a complication of uterine fibroids: a retrospective descriptive study. Journal of Obstetrics and Gynecology, 2009, vol.29, no.8, pp.732–736.

[38] Fletcher HM, Wharfe G. Intestinal obstruction and thromboembolism in a postmenopausal woman with large calcified fibroids. Journal of Obstetrics and Gynecology, 2008, vol.28, no.7, pp.754–755.

[39] Olive DL, Pritts EA. Fibroids and reproduction. Seminars in Reproductive Medicine, 2010, vol.28, no.3, pp. 218–227.

[40] Olive DL. The surgical treatment of fibroids and infertility. Seminars in Reproductive Medicine, 2011, vol.29, no.2, pp.113–123.

[41] Duhan N. Current and emerging treatments for uterine myoma — an update. International Journal of Women's Health, 2011, vol.3, pp.231–241.

[42] Lupattelli T, Clerissi J, Basile A, et al. Treatment of uterine fibromyom with bilateral uterine artery embolization: state of the art. Minerva Ginecol. 2007; 59(4):427–439.

[43] van der Kooij SM, Bipat S, Hehenkamp WJ, Ankum WM, Reekers JA. Uterine artery embolization versus surgery in the treatment of symptomatic fibroids: a systematic review and metaanalysis. Am J Obstet Gynecol. 2011; 205(4):317.

[44] Moss JG, Cooper KG, Khaund A, et al. Randomised comparison of uterine artery embolisation (UAE) with surgical treatment in patients with symptomatic uterine fibroids (REST trial): 5-year results. BJOG. 2011; 118(8):936–944.

[45] Al-Badr A, Faught W. Uterine artery embolization in an undiagnosed uterine sarcoma. Obstet Gynecol. 2001; 97(5):836–837.

[46] Tulandi T, Sammour A, Valenti D, Child TJ, Seti L, Tan SL. Ovarian reserve after uterine artery embolization for leiomyomata. Ferti Steril. 2002; 178(1):197–198.

[47] Kaump GR, Spies JB. The impact of uterine artery embolization on ovarian function. J Vasc Interv Radiol. 2013; 24(4):459–467.

[48] Vercellini P, Oldani S, DeGiorgi O, Cortesi II, Moschetta M, Crosignani PG. Endometrial ablation with a vaporizing electrode in women with regular uterine cavity or submucous leiomyomas. J Am Assoc Gynecol Laparosc. 1996; 3(4):S52.

[49] Froeling V, Meckelburg K, Schreiter NF, et al. Outcome of uterine artery embolization versus MR-guided high-intensity focused ultrasound treatment for uterine fibroids: long-term results. Eur J Radiol. 2013; 82(12):2265–2269.

[50] Mara M, Horak P, Kubinova K, Dundr P, Belsan T, Kuzel D. Hysteroscopy after uterine fibroid embolization: evaluation of intrauterine findings in 127 patients. J Obstet Gynaecol Res. 2012; 38(5):823–831.

Section 3

Retroperitoneal and Retrograde Total Laparoscopic Hysterectomy

Chapter 5

Retroperitoneal and Retrograde Total Laparoscopic Hysterectomy – Technique with Three- and Five-millimeter Trocars

Eugenio Volpi, Elisa Peano, Giulia Moggio, Anna Silvia Pertusio,
Paola Ballario and Luca Bernardini

Additional information is available at the end of the chapter

http://dx.doi.org/10.5772/61649

Abstract

In this chapter, we describe total laparoscopic hysterectomy (TLH) using retroperitoneal and retrograde technique: it combines the retroperitoneal coagulation of the uterine artery and the retrograde approach to the pelvic organs, as in oncological surgeries. We report our experience in applying this modified TLH with 3-mm instruments and without uterine manipulator, in order to demonstrate its safety and feasibility.

Keywords: Laparoscopy, Hysterectomy, Retroperitoneal hysterectomy, Retrograde

1. Introduction

Mini-invasive approaches have successfully been applied to an increasing number of gynecological procedures. Robotics represents now the state of the art in mini-invasive surgeries, especially in the USA, where it is available in many referral centers [1]. In Europe, laparoscopy is much more widely distributed: total laparoscopic hysterectomy (TLH) is, at present, the main alternative to abdominal hysterectomy (TAH) [2]. TLH is associated with less blood loss, shorter hospital stay, and low rate of infection and ileus in comparison to laparotomy. Patients can avoid painful abdominal incision and return more quickly to their activities [3].

Nowadays, the most diffuse technique for TLH involves intrafascial dissection of vascular pedicles and the use of a manipulator for the mobilization of the uterus and the cervix, as

INTECH
open science | open minds

© 2015 The Author(s). Licensee InTech. This chapter is distributed under the terms of the Creative Commons Attribution License (http://creativecommons.org/licenses/by/3.0), which permits unrestricted use, distribution, and reproduction in any medium, provided the original work is properly cited.

described by the French and Finnish schools [2–5]. According to these authors, the transection of the uterine vessels is performed close to the uterus, medially to the ureter, as in conventional TAH. However, endometriosis, intra-ligamentary fibroids, previous pelvic infections and other anatomical variations could make coagulation or dessication of the ascending and descending branches difficult. Moreover, when coagulation is extensively performed, there is an increased risk of ureteral lesions [6–8]. In this chapter, we describe a modified technique of retroperitoneal (dissection of the uterine arteries) and retrograde (dissection of the bladder and vagina) TLH, with the aim to provide optimal control of the ureter and bleeding. The retroperitoneal laparoscopic approach was originally described by Kohler et al. [9] and Roman et al. [10]; the retrograde culdotomy was reported in the 190s by Delle Piane [11], Hudson and Chir [12], and more recently by Bristow et al. [13].

2. Technique

We described the technique of retroperitoneal and retrograde TLH in a previous paper [14]. Hereby, we report the critical steps of the procedure:

1. Patients are positioned in a dorsal lithotomy with legs apart and semi-flexed and the arms tucked at the sides. The monitor is placed between the patient legs or on her left foot if morcellation is foreseen, facing the two surgeons to facilitate an ergonomic working position. The equipment used is simple: a scissor, two grasping forceps, a washing-aspiration 5-mm device, and a 5-mm bipolar coagulation forceps. Recently, the LigaSure™ 5-mm 37-cm (Covidien LF1537) forceps was added to the instrumentation, avoiding the use of disposable scissors. No uterine manipulator is placed in situ.

We usually access the peritoneum by direct trocar insertion [15]. Only patients with story of surgeries are accessed via Palmer point and Verress needle. Five millimeter optics are used. Three 5-mm trocars are placed in the lower abdomen under direct vision, in the usual diamond-shaped position. Variations may be due to the uterine size: if the uterus has a size less than 13 weeks of pregnancy, the procedure can be started with two mini-laparoscopic trocars on the sides, keeping the umbilical and the suprapubic trocar of 5 mm. Only 3-mm grasping forceps and a 3-mm needle holder are used through the side ports.

The first surgical step is isolation of the ureter and of the uterine artery. The assistant surgeon moves medially the utero-ovarian ligament to stretch the broad ligament. The incision is made up to where the broad ligament overlies the iliac vessels, thus allowing to enter into the retroperitoneum. The peritoneum is opened parallel to the infundibulo-pelvic ligament above the crossing, with the external iliac artery taking care to move the ureter on the medial sheet of the peritoneum (Figure 1).

The ureter is then followed till the crossing with the uterine artery. After dissection, the uterine artery is coagulated at its origin from the internal iliac artery (Figure 2).

http://dx.doi.org/10.5772/61649

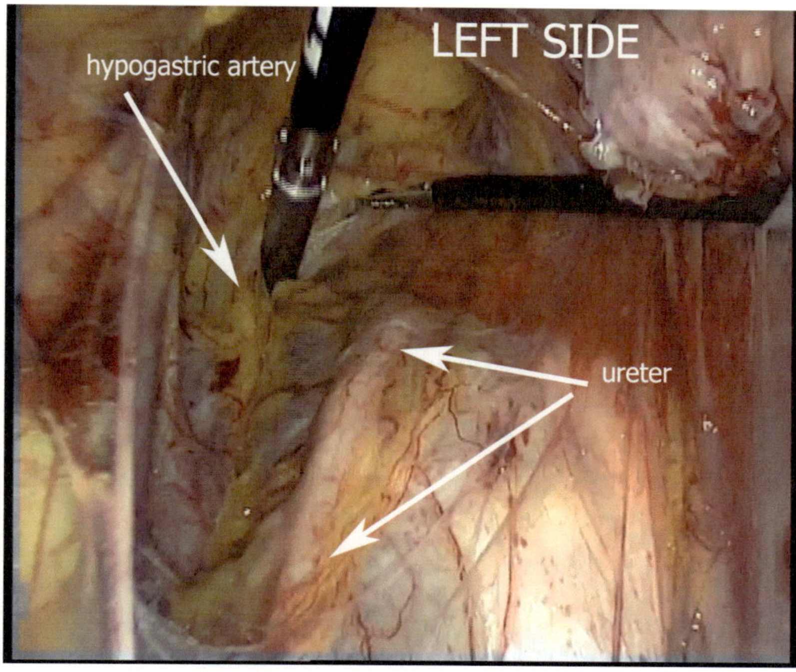

Figure 1. Access to retroperitoneum: the peritoneum is opened parallel to the infundibulo-pelvic ligament; the ureter is identified and followed till uterine artery.

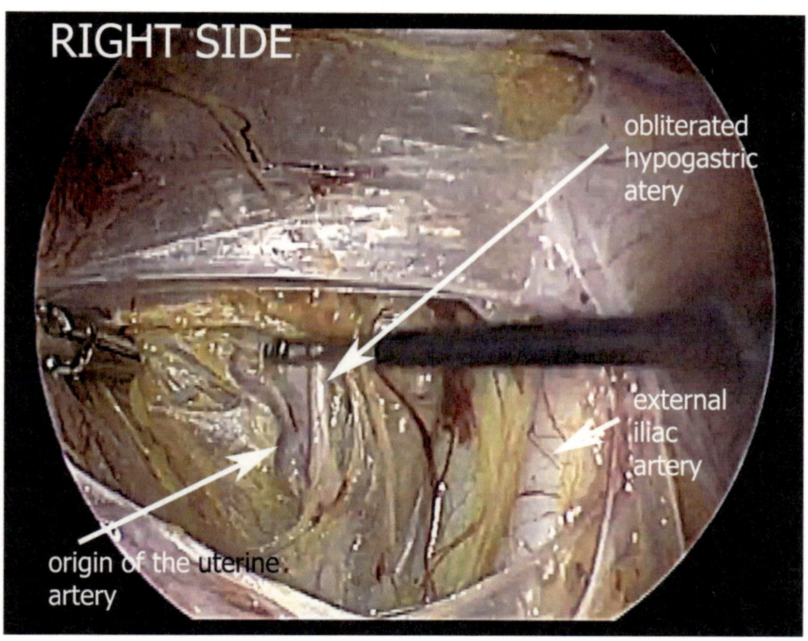

Figure 2. Identification and coagulation of uterine artery at its origin from the internal iliac artery.

We often grasp and coagulate the uterine veins altogether but do not transect the vessels (Figure 3). Since the infundibulo-pelvic ligament is not divided, any bowel interference during the operation is avoided by pulling medially the medial leaf. The same steps are repeated contralaterally.

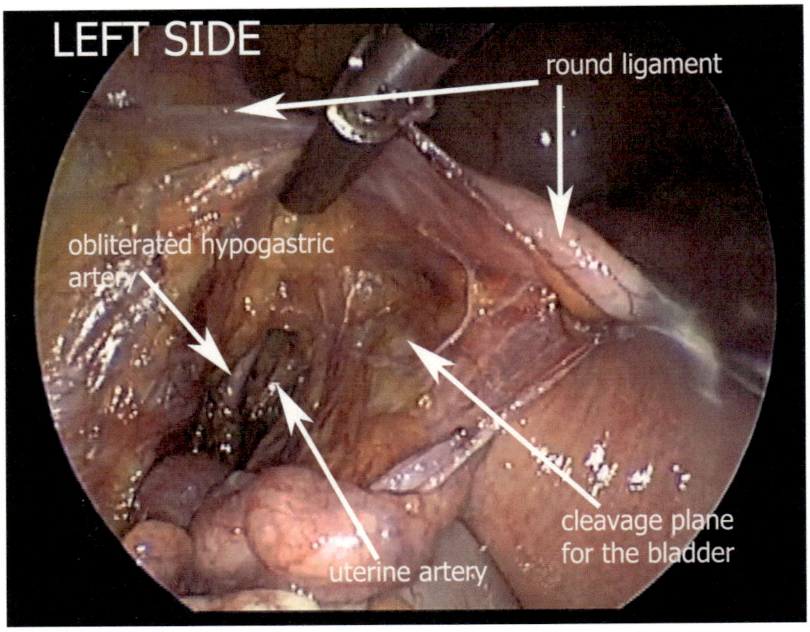

Figure 3. Uterine artery is coagulated but not transected.

2. The round ligament may or may not be divided at this time at the cross with the umbilical artery. Blunt dissection on the vesico-vaginal fascia is performed from the lateral to medial side (Figure 4). The vesico-uterine peritoneal fold is left aside and dissection initiated just distally to the uterine arteries following the pelvic fascia. Dissection is stopped when the white vaginal fornix is reached. At this point, the transection of the round ligament is completed by dividing all the anterior leaf down to the vesico-uterine peritoneal fold, in order to mobilize the bladder from connections to the lower uterine segment. The infundibulo-pelvic or the utero-ovarian ligaments are coagulated and transected after fenestration of the broad ligament with the ureter under control. This approach is important in patients who had previous surgery on the lower uterine segment (e.g. cesarean section).

3. The posterior leaf of the broad ligament is incised toward the posterior vaginal apex and recto-vaginal septum. Now, the uterine artery is coagulated again and transected, being the ureteral course directly visible. Parametrial and uterosacral ligaments may be cut at this time, but usually are controlled by retrograde resection.

By means of a ring forceps, the anterior fornix is exposed by a nurse. This is incised on the bulging of the rings and opened. A vaginal plug is then used to stop CO_2 loss. While the

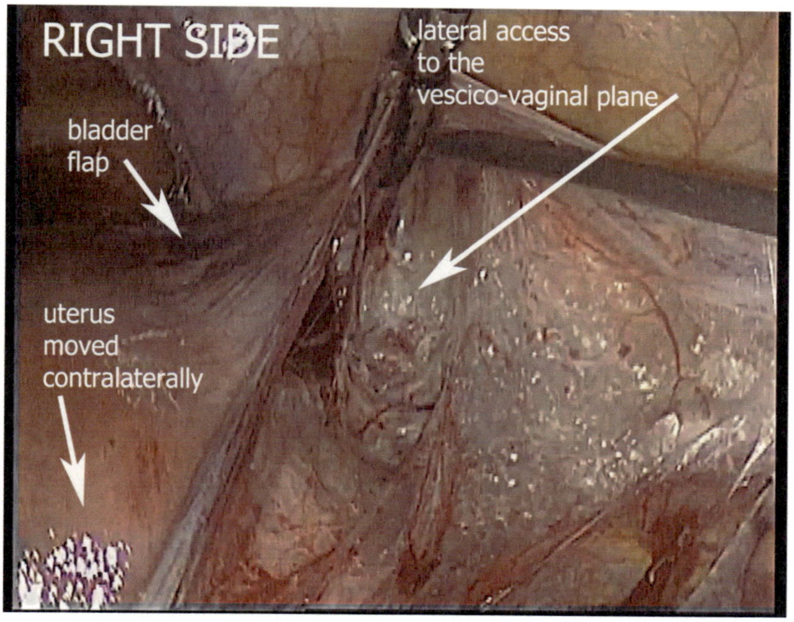

Figure 4. Blunt dissection of vesico-vaginal space.

assistant surgeon grasps and elevates the distal margin of the vagina, the first operator moves proximally the cervical margin of the vagina and starts the retrograde incision of the vagina (Figure 5). This is facilitated by strongly pulling the cervix cranially.

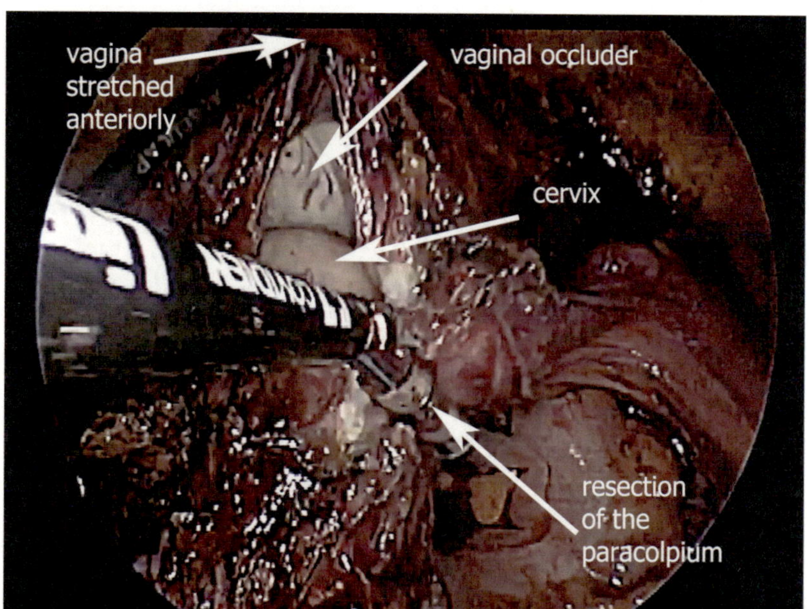

Figure 5. Beginning of retrograde incision of vagina.

Vagina, parametrium and utero-sacral ligaments are severed moving from anterior to posterior aspect and from the vagina toward the cervix, parallel to the ureteral course (Figure 6). During this step, the LigaSure™ forceps is useful since cutting and coagulation may be performed at the same time, while using bipolar forceps and scissors may be more difficult.

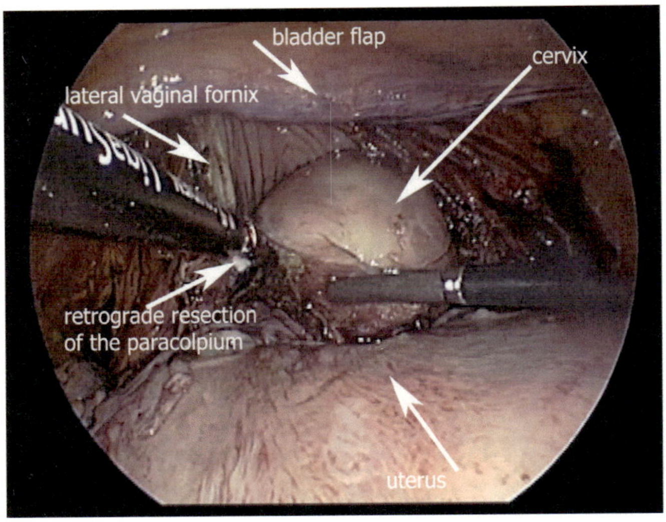

Figure 6. Retrograde dissection of paracolpium.

Classic vaginal morcellation to extract the uterus is performed. In case of very restricted vaginal access, the removal of the uterus is performed by abdominal morcellation.

Finally, the vagina is closed laparoscopically by a running suture using V-lock suture (Covidien) or Caprosyn (Ethicon) (Figures 7 and 8).

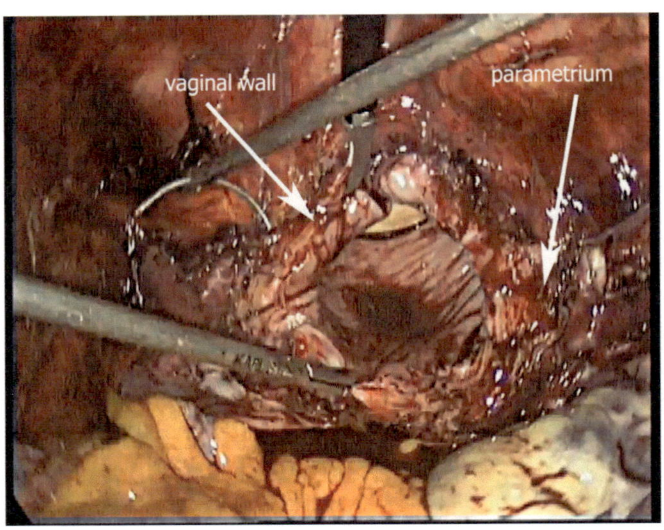

Figure 7. Beginning of vaginal suture.

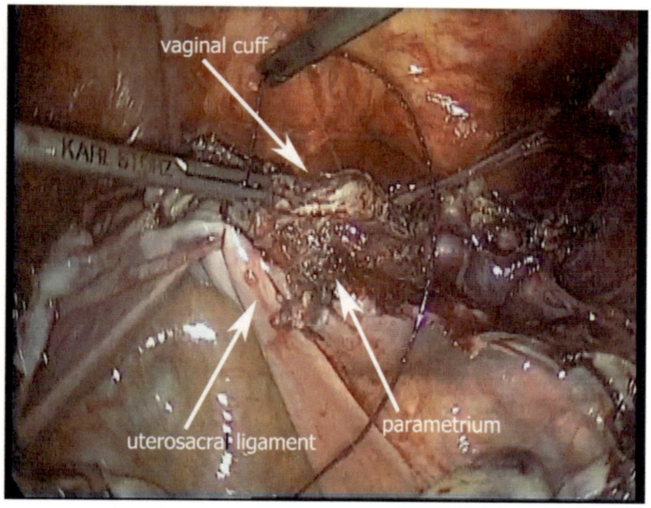

Figure 8. Closure of vaginal cuff.

3. Discussion

We report our experience in applying modified technique for TLH: we combine the retroperitoneal coagulation of the uterine artery and the retrograde approach to the pelvic organs. The retroperitoneal approach has been used mainly during vaginally assisted laparoscopic hysterectomies (VAH) [9, 10, 16–18], while the retrograde bladder dissection and the retrograde culdotomy have been described specifically for laparotomic oncological surgeries [11–13]. To date, just one study by Roman et al. reported the application of a retroperitoneal approach for total laparoscopic hysterectomy in case of enlarged uteri [10].

Up to now, after progressively setting up our technique, we have performed about 1, 000 of these procedures. However, this paper refers to 400 hysterectomies developed in two different hospitals from 2011 to 2013. In our experience, about 94% of hysterectomies can be performed laparoscopically, even if a limitation at 22-week size of the uterus is admitted. Moreover, our experience is reproducible with 3-mm trocars: in these cases, the size of the uterus has been limited to 13-week uterus. We think about the 3-mm experience simply as a scaling down from a previous experience with two 10-mm and two 5-mm trocars: surgical steps and operating time were the same.

We observed a low rate of complications. We registered two ureteral fistulas (0.5% in the last 3 years). The first fistula is a complication due to a very large (12 cm) infraligamentary fibroid: the pelvic ureter beyond uterine artery was longer than usual for the presence of the myoma and so dissection resulted in excessive devascularization. It was managed by re-implantation. The second occurred 16 days after surgery and it was managed by stenting. Both complications were late, at least after 10 days from surgical procedure. Six patients had bladder injury. The lesion was sutured laparoscopically and the patients dismissed on the 3rd day with the catheter in situ. When the patients came back after 1 week of follow-up, the catheter was removed.

The rate of urologic complications observed in our experience may be justified by the absence of selection of the patients except for uterine size and is in agreement to that reported by similar studies using retroperitoneal approach [8–10, 20–22].

We also observed four cases of vaginal cuff dehiscence: this rate is similar to that of the literature.

Our results, in terms of operative time, mean blood loss, mean hospital stay and complications, based on about 400 cases, are comparable to those reported by most centers where laparoscopic hysterectomy is routinely performed according to the classic technique (intrafascial dissection and constant use of uterine manipulator) [9, 10, 23, 24].

Kohler et al. [9] demonstrated full safety and clinical advantages of an extraperitoneal technique: they reported optimal isolation, coagulation and transection of uterine artery and constant control of the ureter during the laparoscopic assistance to 267 vaginal hysterectomies. The interruption of blood supply through this approach especially helped the vaginal removal of enlarged uteri, when bleeding generally is a problem in vaginal operations. Seventy percent of these procedures were performed by residents with limited surgical experience; moreover, the use of neither not disposable instruments nor uterine manipulator allowed to reduce financial costs. Chang et al. [17] reported their experience in uterine artery ligation through retrograde tracking of the umbilical ligament: the blood loss (two patients lost >500 mL) was minimal and complication rate very low (two bladder laceration) in 225 laparoscopic-assisted vaginal hysterectomies for myomas or adenomyomas. The average time from identification of the umbilical ligament to ligation of the uterine artery was approximately 10 min and operations were performed by residents with aid of the attending physician. In our experience, the technique to dissect the uterine artery is different, but the time spent is similar.

Roman et al. described more than 50 cases of TLH for large uteri with uterine coagulation at its origin [10]. Their results confirmed that the retroperitoneal approach is feasible and reproducible by gynecological surgeons avoiding laparotomy for enlarged uteri. According to the authors, the key to a successful procedure is to perform the uterine devascularization before any other surgical step on uterus. In their department, one surgeon began practicing this technique and subsequently it was acquired and easily reproduced by others. These data have been confirmed by other authors [16, 17, 21–23].

For beginners, this modified TLH could seem more challenging than traditional intrafascial hysterectomy; nevertheless, it allows a right approach to more complex pelvic pathologies, as endometriosis or cancer, thanks to a progressive confidence with anatomical spaces and tissues. The retroperitoneal approach is, indeed, mandatory for pelvic lymphadenectomy and useful in case of symptomatic fibroids and ovarian cystectomies with severe adhesions [22]. For patients with fixed uterus or endometriosis, the preventive occlusion of the uterine arteries through downstream ureter tracking in the retroperitoneum decreases the risks of bleeding and ureteral injury; this alternative procedure also shortens the operative time and minimizes the conversion rate to laparotomy [18].

http://dx.doi.org/10.5772/61649

In our experience, the uterine manipulator is not useful: the first assistant can easily expose lateral aspect of uterus because it is free at the level of the isthmus. Furthermore, the position of the optics in the umbilicus can be maintained with an enlarged uterus, since the displacement given by manipulator needs that the camera is moved up, toward the xiphisternum. The disadvantage with a larger uterus is that all the movements are bound to the laparoscopic instruments and it may need more skills. The lateral approach to the uterine arteries and the retrograde resection of the vagina are independent from a uterine manipulator. In our opinion, it is in fact a cultural rather than a technical question.

The technique we described unifies for the first time in a single procedure different surgical steps already reported. Summarizing:

1. Uterine vessels are coagulated at their origin but not transected; the pararectal space is firstly opened.

2. The bladder is approached from the lateral aspect for a safer dissection, especially when anatomical difficulties are present.

3. The ureter is easily visible during the whole procedure.

4. The retrograde circular colpotomy is performed after minimal preparation of the recto-vaginal septum being safely far from the ureter.

5. The whole surgery can be performed without uterine manipulator and with reusable instruments, decreasing the costs.

Oncological preparation of the surgical field as done during the creation of the Latzko's space (preparation of the uterine arteries at their origin) might seem excessive; nevertheless, post-operative course of our patients shows no differences with traditional TLH.

Moreover, our approach includes all the advantages of laparoscopic surgery such as magnification of the anatomy and pathology; access to the uterine vessels, vagina, rectum, and lymph nodes; better exposure of ureter; and achievement of clots drainage and hemostasis [24, 25].

In conclusion, our modified technique of extraperitoneal and retrograde laparoscopic hysterectomy, even if at first appears challenging, allows routine approach to almost all hysterectomies and can offer great prospects for research in gynecological surgery.

Author details

Eugenio Volpi, Elisa Peano, Giulia Moggio, Anna Silvia Pertusio, Paola Ballario and Luca Bernardini*

*Address all correspondence to: volpi.e@ospedale.cuneo.it

Department of Obstetrics and Gynecology, Ospedale S. Croce e Carle, Cuneo, Italy

References

[1] Soto E, Lo Y, Friedman K, Soto C, Nezhat F, Chuang L, Gretz H. Total hysterectomy versus da Vinci robotic hysterectomy: Is using the robot beneficial ? J Gynecol Oncol 2011;22(4):253–9. doi: 0.3802/jgo.2011.22.4.253.

[2] Wattiez A, Cohen SB, Selvaggi L. Laparoscopic hysterectomy. Curr Opin Obstet Gynecol 2002 Aug;14(4):417–22.

[3] Canis M, Botchorishvili R, Ang C, Rabischong B, Jardon K, Wattiez A, Mage G. When is laparotomy needed in hysterectomy for benign uterine disease ? J Minim Invasive Gynecol 2008;15:38–43. doi: 10.1016/j.jmig.2007.09.003.

[4] Kauko M. New techniques using the ultrasonic scalpel in laparoscopy. Curr Opin Obstet Gynecol 1998;10(4):303–305.

[5] Einarsson JI, Suzuki Y. Total laparoscopic hysterectomy: 10 steps toward a successful procedure. Rev Obstet Gynecol 2009;2(1):57–64.

[6] Ostrzenski A, Radolinski B, Ostrzenska KM. A review of laparoscopic ureteral injury in pelvic surgery. Obstet Gynecol Surv 2003;58(12):794–9.

[7] Brummer THI, Jalkanen J, Fraser J, Heikkinen AM, Kauko M, Makinen J, Seppala T, Sjoberg J, Tomas E, Harkki P. FINHYST, a prospective study of 5279 hysterectomies. Complications and their risk factors. Hum Reprod 2011;26(7):1741–51. doi: 10.1093/humrep/der116.

[8] Garry R, Fountain J, Brown J, Manca A, Mason S, Sculpher M, Napp V, Bridgman S, Gray J, Lilford R. Evaluate hysterectomy trial: a multicentre randomised trial comparing abdominal, vaginal and laparoscopic methods of hysterectomy. Health Technol Assess 2004;8:26, 1–140.

[9] Kohler C, Hasenbein K, Klemm P, Tozzi R, Schneider A. Laparoscopic-assisted vaginal hysterectomy with lateral transection of the uterine vessels. Surg Endosc 2003;17:485–90.

[10] Roman H, Zanati J, Friederich L, Resch B, Lena E, Marpeau L. Laparoscopic hysterectomy of large uteri with uterine artery coagulation at its origin. JSLS 2008;12:25–9.

[11] Delle Piane G. Surgery in the modern treatment of ovarian carcinoma. Fifth World Congress of Gynecology and Obstetrics. Sydney: Butterworth, 1967:473–96.

[12] Hudson CN, Chir M. A radical operation for fixed ovarian tumors. J Obstet Gynaecol Br Cwlth 1968;75:1155–6.

[13] Bristow RE, del Carmen MG, Kaufman HS, Montz FJ. Radical oophorectomy with primary stapled colorectal anastomosis for resection of locally advanced epithelial ovarian cancer. J Am Coll Surg 2003;197(4):565–74.

[14] Volpi E, Bernardini L, Angeloni M, Cosma S, Mannella P. Retroperitoneal and retrograde total laparoscopic hysterectomy as a standard treatment in a community hospital. Eur J Obstet Gynecol Reprod Biol 2014;172:97–101. doi: 10.1016/j.ejogrb.2013.10.013.

[15] Volpi E, Sismondi P. Semi-open direct trocar insertion method for induction of pneumoperitoneum at laparoscopy. Gynaecol Endosc 2002;11:197–200.

[16] Shutz K, Possover M, Merker A, et al. Prospective randomized comparison of laparoscopic-assisted vaginal hysterectomy (LAVH) with abdominal hysterectomy (AH) for the treatment of the uterus weighing > 200g. Surg Endosc 2002;16:121–5.

[17] Chang WC, Torng PL, Huang SC et al. Laparoscopic-assisted vaginal hysterectomy with uterine artery ligation through retrograde umbilical ligament trafficking. J Minim Invasive Gynecol 2005;12:336–42.

[18] Hsu WC, Chang WC, Huang SC, Sheu BC, Torng PL, Chang DY. Laparoscopic-assisted vaginal hysterectomy for patients with extensive pelvic adhesions: a strategy to minimise conversion to laparotomy. Aust New Zea J Obstet Gynaecol 2007;47:230–34.

[19] Sinha R, Sundaram M, Nikam YA, Hegde A, Mahajan C. Total laparoscopic hysterectomy with earlier uterine artery ligation. J Minim Invasive Gynecol. 2008;15(3):355–9. doi: 10.1016/j.jmig.2008.01.012.

[20] Pan HS, Ko ML, Huang LW, Chang JZ, Hwang JL, Chen SC. Total laparoscopic hysterectomy (TLH) versus coagulation of uterine arteries (CUA) at their origin plus total laparoscopic hysterectomy (TLH) for the management of myoma and adenomyosis. Minim Invasive Ther Allied Technol 2008;17(5):318–22. Erratum in: Minim Invasive Ther Allied Technol 2008;17(6):370.

[21] Gol M, Kizilyar A, Eminoglu M. Laparoscopic hysterectomy with retroperitoneal uterine artery sealing using LigaSure: Gazi hospital experience. Arch Gynecol Obstet 2007;276:311–4.

[22] Reich H. Total laparoscopic hysterectomy: indications, techniques and outcomes. Curr Opin Obstet Gynecol 2007;19:337–44.

[23] Nieboer TE, Johnson N, Lethaby A, Tavender E, Curr E, Garry R, van Voorst S, Mol BWJ, Kluivers KB. Surgical approach to hysterectomy for benign gynaecological disease. Cochrane Database Syst Rev 2009;8(3). doi: 10.1002/14651858.CD003677.

[24] Ostrzenski A. A systematic arrangement of laparoscopic total abdominal hysterectomy: a new technique. J Natl Med Assoc 1999;91:404–9.

[25] Dubuisson JB, De Dycker Y, Yaron M. The retroperitoneal approach in minimally invasive pelvic surgery. Ann NY Acad Sci 2006;1092:187–98.

Section 4

Total Laparoscopic Hysterectomy, Radical Hysterectomy and Pelvic Exenteration for Pelvic Malignancies

Chapter 6

Radical Hysterectomy Techniques — Indications and Complications

Ambrogio P Londero, Serena Bertozzi,
Luca Martella, Giulio Bertola, Giorgio Giorda,
Angelo Calcagno, Arrigo Fruscalzo and Ralph J Lellé

Additional information is available at the end of the chapter

Abstract

Radical hysterectomy is an important surgical procedure in gynecologic oncology. New technologies are changing hysterectomy techniques, and integrated treatments could expand the surgical indications in gynecologic oncology. Minimally invasive (laparoscopic or robotic surgery) radical hysterectomy adoption is slowed by different factors despite the apparent improvement of morbidity outcomes. Moreover, data about oncologic long-term outcomes of minimally invasive radical hysterectomy are relatively sparse, and more research is needed.

Keywords: Radical hysterectomy, Gynecologic oncology, Hyperthermic intraperitoneal chemotherapy (HIPEC), Open surgery, Laparoscopic surgery, Robotic surgery

1. Introduction

Hysterectomy is the surgical removal of the uterus, and it may be total (removal of the body, fundus, and cervix of the uterus) or partial (removal of the uterine body while leaving the cervix intact; also called supracervical). It is the most commonly performed gynecological surgical procedure, and in the majority of cases, it is performed for benign conditions. This procedure in particular could be:

- Subtotal hysterectomy (supracervical): removal of the uterus, leaving the cervix in situ.
- Total hysterectomy: complete removal of the uterus and cervix.

INTECH
open science | open minds

© 2015 The Author(s). Licensee InTech. This chapter is distributed under the terms of the Creative Commons Attribution License (http://creativecommons.org/licenses/by/3.0), which permits unrestricted use, distribution, and reproduction in any medium, provided the original work is properly cited.

- Radical hysterectomy: complete removal of the uterus, cervix, upper vagina, and parametrium. Indicated for cancer. Lymph nodes, ovaries, and fallopian tubes are also usually removed in this situation.

This chapter would relate about radical hysterectomy performed by abdominal way, taking into consideration also robotic techniques. This technique is performed in cases of malignant diseases affecting the uterus.

2. Indications

Radical hysterectomy is still the treatment of choice for women with early stage cervical cancer [1, 2]. However, modified radical hysterectomy or total hysterectomy is indicated in uterine and ovarian cancers as well. Also in these cases, lymph nodes, ovaries, and fallopian tubes are usually removed as well as the omentum and peritoneum in some circumstances.

3. Historical notes

Radical hysterectomy with pelvic lymphadenectomy is a key intervention in gynecologic oncology, proposed by Wertheim (without lymphadenectomy) for the first time in 1898, and has gradually been enriched by numerous contributions until the excision of pelvic lymph nodes proposed by Meigs (1951) [3].

There is also a vaginal radical hysterectomy, not particularly diffused. That is performed only in a few centers even though the mortality from the beginning was much lower than the laparotomy. Schuchardt had the idea to offer this type of surgery against cervix carcinoma; Schauta codified and made him known to scientific societies; Amreicht took care of the details.

4. Preoperative preparation of the patient

The staging of cervical cancer, and thus the decision for surgery versus radiation, is based on the subjective impression of a clinical investigation. Cystoscopy and sigmoidoscopy are only useful for advanced tumors. In such tumors, however, the primary combined radiotherapy with chemotherapy is usually the treatment of choice.

An intravenous pyelogram is necessary to show or exclude urinary tract duplication or other anomalies. Furthermore, the International Federation of Gynecology and Obstetrics (FIGO) staging system can only be specified if the result of the intravenous pyelogram is known. In fact, a renal accumulation corresponds to a clinical stage IIIB.

Computed tomography scan and magnetic resonance imaging are not necessary and do not provide any additional information. However, a computed tomography scan showing the renal apparatus by contrast medium represents a valid alternative to intravenous pyelogram.

A bowel preparation with polyethylene glycol (PEG) is not necessary and represents only an additional burden on the patient. Before the operation, antibiotic prophylaxis is performed, for example, 2 g cefoxitin intra venous at induction of anesthesia and again two hours after surgery begins, since cephalosporins have only a short half-life of approximately 45 min. Antibiotic prophylaxis should be continued for up to 24 h.

The patient is always examined again under anesthesia, by vaginal (index finger) and rectal (middle finger) exploration.

In case of endometrial cancer, the histologic information obtained from endometrial biopsy (fractioned dilatation and curettage or hysteroscopy and biopsies) usually is sufficient to plan definitive treatment. Other useful tests such as computed tomography, magnetic resonance imaging, and positron emission tomography are used to evaluate extrauterine disease.

5. Abdominal hysterectomy

5.1. Operators and operative theater

Not least, radical hysterectomies have become less frequent, even on larger hospitals; each of these operations should be used for training. With proper instruction, this is not associated with an increased risk for the patient, possibly with a prolongation of the duration of surgery.

After anesthesia induction, the patient is placed in a supine position. Three doctors are involved in the operation. The forming and ultimately for the operation responsible physician is the right of the patient and demonstrates each operation step on one side, including the specific steps below abdominal opening described. In the beginning, it is recommended that the preparation of the uterus is performed on the ipsilateral side and the pelvic lymphadenectomy on the contralateral side. Over time, however, all phases of operation should be practiced from all angles. The third doctor observes the operation and is relieved by the use of the self-holding frame, which is shown to increase its concentration. Depending on the level of training, he may be involved in some operation steps, e.g., abdominal opening and closure.

5.2. Abdominal opening

5.2.1. Morley laparotomy modified by Lellé

Before skin disinfection (as precaution until the level of the nipples) and sterile covering, the incision site is drawn. The Morley interiliac transverse incision [4] is a slightly curved bisiliac cross section. Suitable for marking is the concave side of the Toussaint ruler [5].

Using a scalpel (number 10 or 21), the abdominal skin is incised superficially. The incision can be carried so superficially that there is no bleeding and the subcutaneous fatty tissue is not yet visible. The wound margins are tight and it is possible to continue the incision with the needle electrode of the argon plasma coagulation. Minor bleeding can be directly stopped with the coagulator. If major bleeding occurs, it is coagulated using a modified bipolar forceps with a DeBakey grip panel. The skin edge should not be violated. In the area of the wound, the inferior superficial epigastric veins are coagulated before cutting.

After incision, the fascia is raised with a Péan and further cut across by argon plasma coagulation.

Now, the superficial connective tissue of the right lateral rectus muscle is opened. The Army-Navy hook lifts the edge of the rectus muscle slightly. The deep inferior epigastric artery and vein are identified and disposed by two Overholt clamps. The ligature is like all these ligatures with the strength Polysorb™(Lactomer glycolide/Lactide copolymer coated with caprolactone and calcium stearoyl lactylate) 4-0, although this is a relatively small thread. However, the tensile strength of the material is much higher than polyglactin 910 (Vicryl™). Crucial here is that the node is right and not "falling out." All ligatures are attached by a Pean to a terminal (this is valid in all steps in this description).

Rarely, it may happen that the epigastric vessels are not identified on a side. If the vessels are not even clearly identified, one can instead perform the following procedure: the rectus muscle pitched up by the fingers and cut coming from the lateral until the epigastric vessels are visible. These are then ligated as described above.

The rectus muscle is divided from the peritoneum by the fingers. The Army-Navy retractor is inserted under the muscle and raised. Here, it must be ensured that the peritoneum was not opened accidentally because the intestine can be injured. The rectus muscle is slowly cut by argon plasma coagulation. Bleeding muscle fibers are taken by a Russian forceps and coagulated. Then hemostasis is carefully performed.

The peritoneum is opened best starting from the left, especially if one has gone through appendectomy before, and adhesions may exist on the right side. The peritoneum is lifted with two surgical forceps and opened with a scalpel until the index and middle fingers can be inserted without problems. Above these fingers, with the help of argon plasma coagulation, the peritoneum is fully opened.

5.2.2. Median laparotomy

After skin disinfection by povidone-iodine or clorexidine and sterile covering, the skin is cut along a line which connects the umbilicus to the middle point of the pubis. In fact, this incision is usually called subumbilicus-pubic incision. After the skin, the different abdominal layers are ordinately cut as follows: subcutaneous tissue, linea alba connecting the two rectum muscles of the abdomen, and finally peritoneum, paying attention not to injure the intra-abdominal organs.

This kind of incision could be performed even on a previous median laparotomic scar, obviously more carefully due to the probable presence of adhesions. Moreover, during surgical intervention, it may be elongated from the umbilicus until the xiphoid process if required.

5.3. Exploration of abdominal cavity

First, with the aid of a 50 ml syringe filled with 30 ml of saline, a Douglas lavage is performed and the collected sample is sent for cytological examination. Then the entire abdominal cavity is carefully and systematically examined by visual inspection and/or palpation. In this occasion, the abdominal wall can be lifted with a large Langenbeck hook. In particular, the following structures should be evaluated: the right and the left diaphragm, liver, gallbladder, spleen, stomach (check correct nasogastric tube placement), pancreas, kidney, omentum (also visual inspection), and colon frame down to the rectum. Particularly important is the assessment of the para-aortal region. This can be best assessed from the left side if the mesenteric root is pushed to the side.

The cecum and optionally the appendix are inspected. Then the small bowel is inspected from the ileocecal valve (beginning of the small bowel) down to the mesenteric root. In fact, the small bowel is drawn between the forefinger and thumb and until the Treitz ligament is reached.

Now the surgical retractor is used (Omni-Tract or Bookwalter surgical retractor), leaving the bowel in the abdominal cavity. Then, a kocher clamp is placed in the middle of each utero-ovarian ligament. This must be taken to ensure that uterine veins and arteries will not be accidentally injured. Finally, the two kocher clamps are pulled with one hand, and with the other hand, the cervical length, the parametrium, the paracolpos, and the pelvic lymph nodes are assessed. Also, the peritoneal surfaces and the adnexa are here carefully inspected.

5.4. Preparation of operative field

The Omni-Tract™ surgical retractor is mounted on the top left of Maquet™ table. Although it is a cross section of "Wishbone," it is placed along frames. Four Mayo hooks are used. The two caudal hooks must be taken with caution especially in thin patients that no pressure is exerted on the femoral nerve. During the procedure, the position is reviewed regularly, taking care that the hooks are not pressed posteriorly.

A damp cloth belly, which was folded and rolled into thirds, is placed in each of the right and left para coli rule gutter. The intestine is wrapped with an open cloth and pushed cranially, with one end of cloth in the para-coli. If required, a long reel is inserted transversely. The cranial Mayo hook Omni-Tracts™can be set slightly posteriorly to fix the towels. The big or small flexible window hook should preferably not be used to save space.

5.5. Preparative assessment of operability

The following preparation is exclusively sharply with small steps using the Stevens scissors and Münster forceps, the latter for bipolar coagulation. The Münster forceps is a modified DeBakey forceps with the typical grip profile and bipolar coagulation capability. Forceps is used both for preparation and for coagulation. The coagulation is controlled via a footswitch.

First, the peritoneum is opened in the lateral pelvic area to the right, and the round ligament is exposed. The incision is carried away from the bladder reflection fold. An Overholt clamp is passed under the round ligament and is placed far laterally; then by means of two clamps, the round ligament is held, cut, and tied by a 4-0 Polysorb™ ligature. All of the following ligatures are immediately cut off by the assistant doctor. Then, using the closed scissors and the closed forceps, the pararectal space is opened ("chopstick technique").

Usually, here the ureter is already visible, which is fixed at the medial peritoneal leaf. If the ureter is not clearly visible, you can always palpate it well by scanning the medial peritoneal leaf between the thumb and forefinger.

Index and middle fingers are following introduced pararectal to continue to open the space of the sacrum cave. With the help of a DeBakey forceps, the bladder peritoneum is raised caudally to the right. One sees here a discrete indentation of the bound tissue. Here you go once again with the "chopstick technique" in order to open the paravescical space. With the fingers, the space is stretched again.

Often you can see here already that lateral umbilical ligament, that represents the terminal ramifications of the internal iliac artery. Sometimes one has the impression that it could be the ureter. The ureter is, however, more dorsally and medially visible and is so far caudally never visible because it runs in the bladder pillars. If during this phase of preparation bleeding occurs - usually venous bleeding in pararectal space - it is compressed with a cloth strip and hemostasis is not attempted.

With the index and middle fingers, the parametrium can be palpated and a possible infiltration detected.

The same steps will be executed on the left side.

Then the urinary bladder is sharply dissected from the uterus' anterior wall. The hemostasis is carried out with the Münster bipolar forceps. If strong adhesions exist and the bladder anatomy is unclear, a targeted opening of extraperitoneal bladder is considered to prevent thinning of the detrusor muscle in the trigone and the emergence of a bladder-vaginal fistula [6]. If the bladder is not infiltrated, the operation is continued.

5.6. Pelvic lymphadenectomy

Typically, the operator standing on the right begins with the pelvic lymphadenectomy on the left, so the opposite side of him.

The peritoneum is further cleaved along the para-coli channel cephalad, just caudal to the external iliac artery. Either a Mayo hook Omni-Tract™ is readjusted caudally and slid under the peritoneum or a Roux hook is used by the assistant and pulled caudally.

Cranial iris hooks of Omni-Tract™ are used (corresponding to the heart-shaped Harrington hook), pulling it medially and superiorly.

The ureter crosses the common iliac artery just before its bifurcation and is deported medially from the surgical field.

The resection limits are described in Table 1.

Lateral	Genitofemoralis nerve/iliopsoas muscle
Medial	Internal iliac artery or caudal lateral umbilical ligament
Cranial	Bifurcation of the common iliac artery into the external and internal iliac artery
Caudal	V. circumflex ileum profunda

Table 1. Resection limits of pelvic lymphadenectomy

In detail, the procedure is as follows:

It is only in sharp dissection that the Stevens scissors and Münster forceps are used. Blunt dissection, spreading the tissue with scissors should be avoided since significant leverage forces occur and the tissue is torn violently. In fact, blunt dissection only appears safer than a sharp dissection but it is not.

Hemostasis is always bipolar or done by setting titanium clips. In fact, monopolar coagulation cannot precisely control the coagulation site, and this could lead to damage of important structures.

The fat and the connective tissue are just longitudinal and medial to the genitofemoral nerve split. Here and in the following preparations, it will always work full length of the resection territory described above. Now a blunt instrument is entered between the iliopsoas and external iliac artery or vein with the finger and the vessels are bluntly detached from the muscle. The mobilization is due to the full-length resection described above. Occasionally, a perforator vessel must be coagulated. On the rear wall of the external iliac artery, tissue is dissected using Stevens scissors and Münster forceps laterally to medially.

The external iliac artery is undermined and a Lidhaken (vein retractor after Cushing) is used. The tissue is further dissected until the entire artery is exposed. Subsequently, the preparation of the external iliac vein analog proceeds.

For the part of the lymph node dissection, the internal iliac artery serves as the lead structure, which expires lateral to the umbilical ligament. Usually, in this step, the origin of the uterine artery is already visible.

The whole preparation of lymph node and adipose tissue is done in a single block. This procedure should be learned as a systematic preparation.

For small bleeding, the artery or vein can be attempted in a bipolar coagulation with the Münster forceps when vascular stumps are still present. When bleeding comes from the vein, a small titanium clip can be set alternatively. In the presence of greater bleeding, a vessel could be sutured with a 5-0 polypropylene suture (Prolene™) by using a C-1 needle. If necessary, the artery can be briefly turned off by delicate vascular clamps. In the vein, a small Satinsky clamp could be placed tangentially to the vascular injury.

With the help of the Lidhakens, the external iliac vein is slightly raised to mobilize the tissue directly below the vein. The obturator nerve is also shown by sharp dissection and deported with a small dissection of the ventral fat tissue from the nerves. If no macroscopically tangible lymph node metastases are present, the lymph nodes and fatty tissue are removed anterior to the nerve. Caution should be taken in the area of bifurcation of the common iliac vein in the external and internal iliac vein. The latter consists only of a venous plexus, which is easily vulnerable, leading to problematic bleeding.

For the final preparation of the lymph node and adipose tissue, the lead structures are the internal iliac artery and the lateral umbilical ligament. Usually, the origin of the uterine artery can be already identified.

The lymph nodes in the area of the common vessels are separated for histological examination. Should be noted that no or very little tissue is available on the left side, while on right side the lymph nodes and the fatty tissue are located lateral to the common iliac artery.

The common iliac vein lies just posterior to the tissue to be removed. To avoid injury to the vein - a "classic" complication, if the specific anatomy is not sufficiently known to the surgeon - the vein wall should be identified early and prepared within the vascular sheath. Laterally, attention is paid to the protection of the genitofemoral nerve. Using a Breisky hook, the peritoneum is pushed cranially. The tissue is so far mobilized and it may be discontinued cranially with a large titanium clip.

5.7. Para-aortic lymphadenectomy

The role of para-aortic lymphadenectomy as part of a radical hysterectomy is controversial in the treatment of cervix cancer, while in case of stage II corpus carcinoma, the para-aortic lymphadenectomy is indicated.

Follow the right common iliac artery superiorly to the aorta and cut through the peritoneum as far as necessary. Here, the right ureter must be "skipped" during the preparation. This can then be deported easily laterally. For a more extensive lymphadenectomy, the flexible window hook is used, so that all surgeons and assistants have their hands on the preparation and the control of the possible complications. The hook here pushes the duodenal "C" cranially. Again, the sharp dissection is directly on the vessels which is the safest way. A few finger-widths above the aortic bifurcation is the origin of the inferior mesenteric artery. The artery is preferably protected so as not to influence negatively the colonic blood supply.

Even more than in the pelvic lymphadenectomy, the procedure of dissecting should be gradually carried on with a careful preparation, bipolar hemostasis, and generous setting of titanium clips. Small venous and arterial bleeding in this region is more severe than in the pelvic lymph node dissection.

5.8. Preparation of the ureter and parametrium

With the help of a caudal Breisky hook, the lateral umbilical ligament is put under train.

The uterine arteries are exposed directly to their end from the internal iliac artery. The end of the uterine artery is remarkably conservative in this case. In fact, after an anatomical study by Roberts and Krishingner [7], the artery was in 42 of 44 cases starting from the internal iliac artery or the lateral umbilical ligament.

The artery is clamped by two Meigs forceps or two Overholt forceps. The ligature is performed with a 4-0 Polysorb™. The remaining uterine stump is secured with a small titanium clip that is located upward of the uterus thread that is cut and fixed with a Péan to set something in train for the subsequent preparation. Now, the uterine vein is identified and clamped through small titanium clips. This avoids accidental tear.

When the anatomy is clear enough and the ureter can be clearly identified, the uterine vessels are prepared up to the point where they cross the ureter. The uterine artery over-crosses the ureter, while the vein rarely in some instances could under-cross the ureter as well.

Now the ureter cephalad from the medial peritoneal sheet is sharply dissected and it is mobilized caudally. Here, the ureter is closed to numerous vessels related to the final part of this area, and it is useful to use bipolar coagulation for coagulation before cutting (do not use in this passage unipolar instruments).

Whenever the anatomical relationships are less clear, the ureter is also dissected as previously, used as referral point and mobilized caudally. During the procedure, the ureter with a lid retractor is pulled cranially, to put it under tension; then the ureter has to be followed caudally with an Overholt clamp. The laterally located tissue is cut between two Overholt clamps and ligated with 4-0 Polysorb™.

During the initial bladder mobilization, it was prepared as well for a non-radical hysterectomy in the midline; the bladder will now be further mobilized laterally, so as to isolate the bladder pillar. After a recent blunt mobilization step with the Overholt clamp, the bladder pillar is withdrawn and ligated. In this step, particular attention must be paid to the fact that the ureter is not to be violated. The closed Overholt is used to perforate the tissue, and the movement is medial and forward. Even in the presence, sometimes, of considerable venous hemorrhage, the preparation must be carried out slowly and subtly.

When the ureter is finally exposed to its confluence point into the bladder, the vaginal mucosa could be exposed by rolling further up the bladder.

5.9. Ovariectomy

If a salpingo-oophorectomy is planned, the peritoneum below the infundibulopelvic ligament is windowed using an Overholt clamp. By previous preparation steps, the ureter is here always very visible and usually cannot be violated. Thanks to two Overholt clamps, the ligament is transected and ligated with 4-0 Polysorb™. The proximal clamp is doubly ligated. When you create the first ligature, the clamp is only slightly opened and closed again. The thread is the same cut off to avoid slipping of the ligature by train on the thread. The thread at the distal stump of the uterus situated downward the infundibulopelvic ligament is first left. The peritoneum is sharp cut toward the uterus, and then the thread is tied around the respective Kocher clamp on the uterus.

If the adnexa are left, first the peritoneum between the ligamentum teres uteri and adnexa toward uterus is cut. Then the peritoneum is windowed below the ovarian ligament and the tube. The two structures are then held through an Overholt clamp. Here, it should be ensured that the clamp is not carried too far on the ovary, to avoid injury and bleeding. As a counter clamp is then used a Kocher clamp. The Overholt clamp is replaced by two ligatures - as described above.

5.10. Rectal dissection

The peritoneum is divided transversely in the Douglas area. It is lateral to the two respective ureters, which, however, now should be completely detached from peritoneal leaf. The uterus is then at a maximum to the front pulled to the symphysis under the hand. With the index and middle finger of the other hand, the rectovaginal spatium is dissected and the rectum is displaced from the vagina. Here, a blunt dissection with moderate pressure is only allowed, since the rectum during this step can be quite injured. However, if necessary, the dissection must be sharp under direct vision and directly closed to the vagina. The vagina is dissected here only so far as for the planned discontinuation of the vaginal cuff is necessary. In fact, too-deep pushing leads to unnecessary bleeding.

5.11. Hysterectomy

With the help of slightly curved Zeppelin clamps, the sacrouterine ligaments on both sides should be cut. Here, the clamps are set as close as possible to the sacrum.

However, one must pay attention especially on the left side so that the rectum is not opened. To suture, use Vicryl size 0 on a CT-2 needle. Caution is advised when CR needles are used ("controlled release," "peel needle") so that the needle does not get lost in the operation area.

Finally, when the vagina is opened, all the threads are gathered using a forceps. Moreover, using long clamps, the tissue is cut and ligated until the uterus is completely settled with the vaginal cuff. The still open vagina is completely closed with a Z-suture.

5.12. Radical hysterectomy classification

Radicality of oncological interventions needs always to be balanced with preservation of functional tissues and organs which can be spared by surgical demolition. That is why not only one type of hysterectomy exists, but a variety of possible interventions based on their surgical extension. As a consequence, a consensus about hysterectomy classification has become of crucial importance in order to standardize the nomenclature and consent of a proper comparison of surgical and oncological outcomes.

In 2008, Querleu and Morrow proposed a new classification of radical hysterectomy based on the lateral extent of resection, which takes also into consideration the eventual nerve preservation and separately divides lymphadenectomy into four levels. In particular, hysterectomy has been then classified as follows [8]:

- Type A: Minimum resection of paracervix.

  The cervix is entirely removed through an extrafascial resection, after transection of the paracervix medially to the ureter and laterally to the cervix itself. A minimal (less than 1 cm in length) resection of the vaginal wall is also performed. Indications of this type of hysterectomy are the radical excision of early invasive cancers, as well as the palliative debulking of advanced cancers in a multidisciplinary setting.

- Type B: Transection of the paracervix at the ureter.

  The paracervix is transected at the level of the ureteral tunnel, sparing the caudal neural component of the paracervix caudal to the deep uterine vein, after partial resection of the uterosacral and vesicouterine ligaments. The vagina is resected at least 1 cm from the cervix or from the tumor. These type of hysterectomy results are also indicated for early stage cancers. This procedure may include (B2) or not (B1) paracervical and iliac lymphadenectomy.

- Type C: Transection of paracervix at junction with internal iliac vascular system.

  Hysterectomy is performed through transection of the uterosacral ligament at the rectum, transection of the vesicouterine ligament at the bladder, complete mobilization of both ureters, and vagina resection for about 15-20 mm from the cervix or tumor. This kind of procedure may be performed with (C1) or without (C2) nerve preservation. This intervention is indicated for advanced stage tumors which may be treated with radical intention.

- Type D: Laterally extended resection.

  This kind of hysterectomy consists of the resection of the entire paracervix at the pelvic sidewall (C1), along with the exposure of the sciatic nerve and the resection of hypogastric vessels and vessels which arise from the internal iliac system and reach the lateral part of the paracervix (inferior gluteal vessels, internal pudendal vessels, and obturator vessels). This procedure may additionally be accompanied by resection of the adjacent fascial or muscular structures (C2). In any case, this intervention is rarely performed and is usually part of an ultraradical operation known as pelvic exenteration.

Moreover, lymphadenectomy has been classified based on four levels as follows:

- Level 1: External and internal iliac lymph nodes;
- Level 2: Common iliac lymph nodes (including presacral);
- Level 3: Aortic infra-mesenteric lymph nodes;
- Level 4: Aortic infrarenal lymph nodes.

5.13. Hemostasis and drainage

Hemostasis occurs only after the pelvis is washed extensively. Hereby, the major bleeding will be immediately apparent. After washing, the entire pelvis is compressed with a dry belly cloth. First, the deposition stump of the adnexa or the infundibulopelvic ligament needs to be checked and then the vaginal surgical margins. If necessary, hemostasis is done again with CT-2 or CT-1 Vicryl 0.

The rest of the bleeding is stopped by bipolar coagulation. In case of diffused venous bleeding, stitches are preferably done with 4-0 Vicryl on SH needle.

Special care is often necessary for the hemostasis in the area of the bladder pillar or distal ureter. The smallest is the probability of injury of the ureter, if it is explicitly stitched. In fact, the ureter can be detected by palpation up into the bladder.

Since the peritoneum is completely left open, a drainage of the pelvis is not mandatory [9] and only makes sense if no complete hemostasis was achieved; otherwise, a complete hemostasis should always be sought.

If it is decided for a drainage, a Robinson drainage or better a 10-mm-wide Jackson-Pratt drainage should be taken into consideration. For this, the skin is incised laterally with a scalpel number 11. With an Overholt clamp, the abdominal wall is perforated from the outside inward and the drainage is pulled through from the inside to the outside. For the attachment, a polypropylene suture is used (e.g., Seralene™). Braided threads as Vicryl or Ethibond are less suitable because of their wick effect.

5.14. Suprapubic bladder catheter

By means of the transurethral catheter, the bladder is retrograde filled with saline. Then the sleeve 10 Ch (Charrieres, also known as French Grade (FG): 1 Ch = 1/3 mm diameter) is introduced. Silicone catheter is then inserted in the suprapubic, while with the other hand, the bulging bladder is covered, perforating the bladder. The balloon is filled with 3 ml of saline (at a 12 Ch catheter balloon 5 ml). With pressure on the bladder, it is checked whether the liquid is discharged from the catheter. At the same time, the balloon can be checked and thus the correct location is also reviewed. The transurethral catheter is opened again. At the end of the operation, the transurethral catheter is removed.

5.15. Transposition of the ovaries (in case of pelvic radiotherapy)

Considering the ureter course, the peritoneum is medial to the infundibulopelvic ligament (suspensory ligament). Further severed and isolated the adnexa, in the area of vascular stump two large titanium clips are left. Thereby, the adnexa are shifted upward in women that could necessitate pelvic radiotherapy. By using 4-0 Vicryl on an SH needle on a long needle holder, the adnexa are mounted as high as possible on the lateral peritoneum of the para-coli rule gutters.

The aim is that the ovaries are placed above the promontory; that is the usual radiation limit. With the help of another 4-0 suture, the lateral peritoneal gap is closed. If by mistake a vessel of the infundibulopelvic ligament is injured and cannot be secured by hemostasis, the adnexa must be removed for safety's sake, to prevent re-bleeding.

Figure 1 shows the situs at the end of the operation.

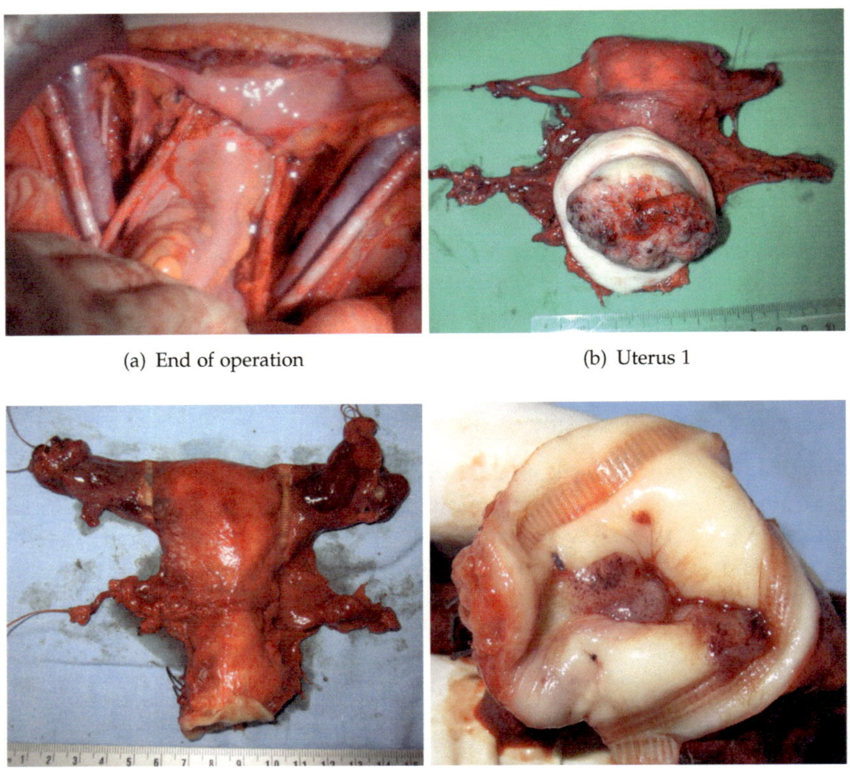

(a) End of operation

(b) Uterus 1

(c) Uterus 2

(d) Cervix with tumor

Figure 1. Figures showing the end of operation

5.16. Abdominal cavity closure

Although the completeness of abdominal swabs and instruments is checked by the nurse, before closure, the abdominal wall of the abdomen is scanned as a precaution.

The table is tilted so that the legs are slightly lifted. An abdomen cloth is laid over the intestine; if necessary, in addition, a flexible blade is used. The fascial corner is pulled using a Roux hook. One last time, it is ensured that the severed muscle bellies and the deposition sites of the epigastric vessels are free from bleeding. The abdominal wall is closed by continuous suture with Biosyn™(thickness of 1 to a 150- cm-long thread that is embedded as a loop in the needle). The needle is guided either by hand, since the needle tip is blunt (pp = "protect point"), or with the Russian forceps. It is important that plenty of tissue is taken, especially in the area of the fascial corner. Otherwise, the rectus muscle or the peritoneum is not combined well. In the center line, one of the two threads is immediately cut at the needle; then the needle is punched for the last time and a knot is done.

The needle is now tied and the thread ends completely removed. At this point, at least six or, better, eight knots must be placed. Biosyn™threads are unlike PDS™threads that lessen the chances of thread "breaks." A second suture is placed starting from the contralateral fascial corner.

Finally, a thread end of the two seams is knotted together in each case. The subcutaneous tissue is checked for blood dryness. The skin is closed by intradermic suture with 5-0 Biosyn™C-13 needle. Instead of a patch association, wide Steri-Strips are stuck in the wound direction.

5.17. Postoperative patient monitoring

The antibiotic (cefoxitin) is added over 24 h and then discontinued. A stomach probe is not required. Once the patient is fully awake, she is allowed to drink and immediately take light food. A gradual approach is not required.

Early mobilization is very important, however, the patient receives a thrombosis prophylaxis with low-molecular-weight heparin in a sufficiently high dose.

The currently inserted Jackson-Pratt drainage is removed after 24 or 48 hours when the postoperative coagulation conditions have stabilized. On the sixth postoperative day, the sovra-pubic catheter is disconnected and the bladder training is started.

The patient can be discharged on the seventh postoperative day, provided that a good home care and short-term medical monitoring are guaranteed. If there is still residual urine at this time, the patient either learns self-catheterization or will be dismissed with a horizontal sovra-pubic catheter.

5.18. Intraoperative and postoperative complications

The main intraoperative complications are ureteral laceration, rectal injury, main arteries or vein injury, and eventual bladder laceration (if not opened intentionally).

The main postoperative complications could be hemorrhage, wound infection, urine retention, ureter stricture, and lymphedema.

In addition, the nerve-sparing radical hysterectomy was introduced with the intent to spare autonomic nerves and in particular bladder function but not compromising surgical radicality [2].

In general, open surgery compared to laparoscopic approach seems to be more prone to have operative complications and stump recurrence [10]. Furthermore, the laparoscopic approach seems to have significant reduction of blood loss and hospital stay [11].

6. The role of laparoscopy in gynecologic oncology and laparoscopic radical hysterectomy

In general, laparoscopic hysterectomy represents very advantageous in comparison with the laparotomic approach, reducing the surgical trauma on pelvic structures with a consequent reduction also in adherence formation, improving postoperative course with a quicker functional recovery (deambulation, canalization, etc.), less pain perception and less drug administration, reduction of the hospitalization length with a quicker recovery of both work activities and social life, and reduction of the postoperative complications.

Common indications for the laparoscopic hysterectomy are uterine myomas and abnormal uterine bleeding but also uterine and cervix carcinoma. However, the laparoscopic approach is not always feasible. Another field of application in gynecologic oncology is ovarian cancer. In fact, laparoscopic staging could be of paramount importance before open surgery. Furthermore, it is considered also the possibility to treat intraperitoneal cancer spread by laparoscopy eventually before intraperitoneal local chemotherapy.

Basically, the laparoscopic technique for hysterectomy differs from previous laparotomic description for the following issues.

6.1. Patient preparation and positioning

After anesthesia induction, women are placed in a dorsal lithotomy position with the arms tucked at the sides. The legs are bent, mildly elevated, and closed in boots in order to allow Trendelenburg during intervention phases.

The insertion of a uterine manipulator for hysterectomy (e.g., uterine HOHL manipulator or uterine Clermont-Ferrand manipulator) through a speculum results very helpful to improve pelvic visibility during the whole intervention. It is of crucial importance to choose the correct size in order to prevent the risk of ureteral injury with larger manipulators and to avoid a bad vaginal fornice delineation in case of smaller ones. The manipulator insertion could be eventually omitted in cases of women who have never had any intercourse or those long-standing treated with testosterone.

6.2. Abdominal entry and trocar placement

Usually the laparoscopic approach is made through four trocars placed as follows:

- 12-mm umbilical trocar, which may be inserted under direct vision or after pneumoperitoneum induction through the Verres needle;
- 5-mm trocar in the right fossa iliaca, lateral to the rectus abdominis muscle 2-cm above and 2-cm medial to the anterior superior iliac spine;
- 12-mm trocar in the left fossa iliaca, lateral to the rectus abdominis muscle 2-cm above and 2-cm medial to the anterior superior iliac spine;
- 5-mm trocar on the left side, 8-cm above and parallel to the lower left trocar site.

During surgery, the uterine manipulator is being pushed upward and to the contralateral side to provide an optimal visualization of the surgical field.

6.3. Uterus removal

After separation of the uterus and cervix from the vaginal apex, the uterus is pulled into the vagina in order to maintain pneumoperitoneum while suturing by laparoscopy. However, it is possible to remove the uterus by vaginal way, closing the vagina with a pneumatic cuff to maintain the pneumoperitoneum. Afterward, it is still possible to close the vagina by laparoscopic approach, but also vaginal approach to close the vaginal apex is feasible.

The vaginal cuff is then sutured, beginning from its distal angle and making sure to include both the vaginal mucosa and the rectovaginal fascia.

Hemostasis is controlled at least three times before port closure.

7. Notes on robotic surgery applied on radical hysterectomy

Robotic surgery represents the new frontier of mini-invasive gynecologic surgery. Along with the same quality and efficacy of traditional surgery, robotic surgery offers all the benefits of mini-invasive surgery, including the absence of big abdominal scars, reduced operative time, reduced blood loss, and reduced postoperative pain. In particular, robots add to the surgical procedure a precision which is not comparable to the other techniques. Moreover, through the great versatility of their instruments, robots may reach very narrow and deep anatomical spaces, being very comfortable especially in the pelvic surgery.

Mini-invasive laparoscopic surgery has experienced a great spread in the gynecologic field at the beginning of the 1990s. Then, robotic surgery represented an evolution of laparoscopic surgery and succeeded in overcoming the limits of laparoscopic surgery itself in reaching anatomically difficult regions.

Surgical robots are constituted by a surgical console and a surgical cart. Sit by the surgical console, the surgeon controls the surgical instruments through some handpieces which are able to complete 360° movements and looks at the operative field through a tridimensional telecamera. The surgical cart is the true robot, obviously localized by the operative table, and usually includes four operative arms.

Surgical instruments are introduced in the abdomen by 8 mm trocars and fixed to the arms of the surgical cart. They are in a continuous technological evolution in order to satisfy surgeons' needs in any surgical discipline. And, most important, they are very versatile and may completely articulate their movements, in order to reach any region of the abdomen, being very advantageous in pelvic surgery or among obese patients, where the intestinal encumbrance reduces the action field.

Actually, all laparoscopic interventions may be converted to robotic ones. Moreover, robotic surgery reduces operative time and consequently anesthesiologic risks and physical stress for the patient. Furthermore, even complex patients may undergo robotic surgery as the CO_2 pressure within the abdomen is lower than those of laparoscopic surgery.

Finally, tridimensional vision helps the surgeon in the identification of nerves, vessels, or ligamentous structures.

7.1. Robotic surgery of the tubes

The first robotic intervention was performed on the tubes. Tubaric surgery, in fact, results particularly difficult especially when they require to be reopened after binding with voluntary sterilization intent. The indication for robotic surgery in this case lays in the evident quality of robotic sutures, which result more simple and safe if performed by robotic instruments.

In particular, tubaric anastomosis requires a suture with very thin reabsorbable threads (6-0 to 8-0), which are used to reconstruct both the muscular and serous layers of the tubes. Moreover, tridimensional vision gives the operator more precision to perform such complex sutures.

7.2. Robotic surgery of uterine myomas

The maximal spread of laparoscopic surgery for the excision of uterine myomas developed during the 1990s, even if the laparotomic approach results were still very frequently used. In fact, laparotomic myomectomy allows a good suture quality and is surely easier to learn while completing the learning curve of a gynecologic surgeon. However, nowadays it has been widely demonstrated that the quality of laparoscopic sutures is comparable to that of laparotomic ones. Moreover, the suture with the robot results in easy and faster execution and thus reduces even the operative and anesthesiologic time.

Thanks to robotic needle holders and to the versatility of their movements, the surgeon can make sutures on the uterus after the myoma excision, even in more layers, in less time and with less blood loss.

7.3. Robotic surgery of endometriosis

Surgery for rectum-vaginal endometriosis is nowadays performed by laparoscopy, and in this case, robotic techniques improve the approach to narrow spaces. The excision of vesical and/or rectal endometriosis is then another fundamental indication for robotic surgery in the gynecologic field, as well as the rectum resection for endometriosis.

Robotic surgery aims to reduce the incidence of stoma formation and to reduce hospitalization time, which results about 5 days, although women result completely autonomous within the second postoperative day.

7.4. Robotic surgery of uterine cancer

In the gynecologic oncologic field, the robotic surgical approach finds nowadays its principal role in the treatment of uterine cancer. In fact, if once this neoplastic disease was treated only by laparotomic incision, now it is possible to operate patients through 3-4 8 mm-sized incisions on their abdominal wall with a consequent increased benefit on their psychophysical wellness.

In this perspective, during the last decade, many authors published their casistic in order to assess feasibility and safety of this procedure in comparison with the traditional approach. And actually, they assessed its feasibility and safety in case of both cervical cancer and endometrial cancer, as well as sarcomas.

Tanks to the tridimensional vision of robot, it is possible to better identify the nerves and to spare them when possible while removing the uterus and consequently to reduce postoperative complications such as urinary retention or urinary incontinence.

In addition, mean operative time results surely inferior than that required for laparotomic hysterectomy and pelvic lymphadenectomy, as well as blood loss and hospitalization time, which for the robotic procedure is about 3 days.

Finally, more rare is the use of robotic approach in case of pelvic recurrences after hysterectomy, but it is not contraindicated.

8. HIPEC in gynecologic oncology

8.1. Definition and epidemiology of peritoneal carcinomatosis in gynecologic malignancies

Peritoneal carcinomatosis is defined as the spread of neoplastic cells in the peritoneal cavity, which usually forms a multitude of nodules on the parietal peritoneum as well as on the visceral peritoneum. It is considered a terminal stage of many solid intra-abdominal tumors, including those of the digestive tract or of the female reproductive system, usually leading to death due to a chronic, progressively worsening, occlusive status [12]. It has a very unfavorable prognosis, and in the literature, the median survival of patients diagnosed with peritoneal carcinomatosis traditionally was not longer than 6 months [13, 14].

Among gynecologic malignancies, epithelial ovarian cancer is recognized to have the most marked propensity for peritoneal involvement. In fact, about 50 to 75% of women with ovarian cancer will develop persistent or recurrent disease [15]. Invasion of the ovarian capsule and dissemination in the peritoneal cavity is the main route by which ovarian carcinoma spreads [15], accounted for about 82% of the cases, whereas in 12% it involves the retroperitoneal lymph nodes [12].

For what concerns uterine cancer, the current literature reported some cases of peritoneal carcinomatosis of endometrial origin, justifying then interest in the loco-regional treatment for such poor prognosis lesions [16, 17].

8.2. Preoperative assessment of peritoneal carcinomatosis

Although the majority of patients affected by gynecologic malignancies undergo computer tomography (CT) scan or magnetic resonance imaging (MRI) or positron emission tomography (FDG/PET-CT) during their pre-recovery period, the diagnosis of peritoneal carcinomatosis remains a great challenge for the radiologist.

In fact, CT scan has a very low sensitivity for nodules smaller than 5 mm, and the 80% of sensitivity is reached in case of CT scan only among patients with diffuse peritoneal carcinomatosis [18, 19].

For what regard FDG/PET-CT, its accuracy results strongly compromised by previous systemic therapies that may lead to an underestimation of disease due to dormant neoplastic foci, as well as to an overestimation of disease because of increased contrast medium uptake in scars or fibrotic areas [20].

In order to standardize peritoneal carcinomatosis assessment, Sugarbaker introduced the Peritoneal Cancer Index (PCI) in 1995 [21], which consists of a score ranging from 0 to 39, depending on both the localization and the size of neoplastic nodules within the peritoneal cavity. In particular, the abdomen is divided into 12 areas (Figure 2), and to any area is given a score considering nodules size as follows:

- 0 no macroscopic disease
- 1 nodules less than 2.5 mm
- 2 nodules between 2.5 mm and 2.5 cm
- 3 nodules greater than 2.5 cm

A second classification exists, introduced by Gilly [22], which is actually more in use only by the French school.

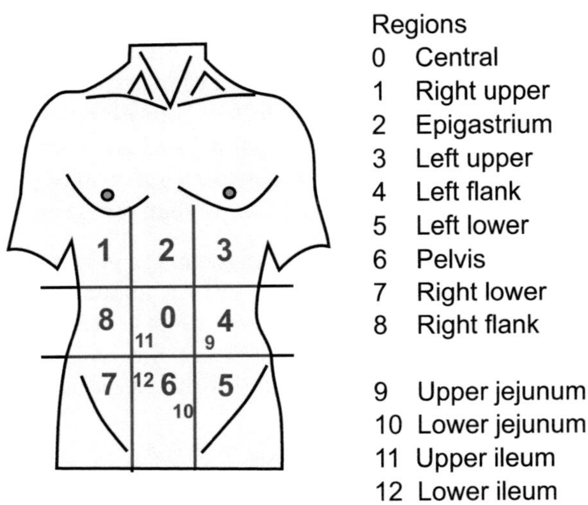

Figure 2. Sugarbaker regions

8.3. Intraoperative assessment of peritoneal carcinomatosis

Intraoperative assessment of peritoneal carcinomatosis is performed before and after CRS. First, peritoneal involvement is evaluated by PCI score as previously described. This is a very important step, because it may predict the radicality of CRS and consequently the possibility to perform the HIPEC. It is possible to perform this step also by laparoscopic approach.

After surgical demolition, residual peritoneal disease is usually measured using the Completeness Cytoreduction Score (CCS), which takes into consideration the residual tumor size as follows:

- CCS0 no macroscopic residual disease
- CCS1 residual disease sized less than 2.5 mm

- CCS2 residual disease between 2.5 mm and 2.5 cm
- CCS3 residual disease greater than 2.5 cm

In case of CCS0-1 HIPEC founds its best indication and is performed with curative intent. CCS2-3 usually contraindicate HIPEC, which in some selected cases is anyway performed but just with a palliative intent, as it is recognized to significantly reduce neoplastic ascitis in the terminal stage disease.

8.4. Cytoreductive Surgery (CRS) and peritonectomy

The surgical procedure of cytoreduction is now well standardized. Sugarbaker's classification is still the reference for abdominal oncologic surgery and goes under the definition of peritonectomy [21]. The surgical procedure was classified according to specific different areas of the abdominal cavity and it has been tailored by Milan's panel workshop, defining:

- Upper Right Peritonectomy: right diaphragmatic peritonectomy with Glisson's capsule dissection; lesser omentectomy, stripping of the omental bursa and cholecystectomy plus gastric antrectomy or total gastrectomy.
- Upper Left Peritonectomy: left diaphragmatic and parietal ritonectomy with splenectomy and greater omentectomy.
- Pelvic Peritonectomy: pelvic parietal peritonectomy, sigmoidectomy, hysterectomy and salpingo-oophorectomy.
- Right Parietal Peritonectomy, right/total colectomy; left parietal peritonectomy.
- Mesenteric implants on visceral surfaces could be removed surgically or by electrosurgical local dissection.

While performing cytoreduction for peritoneal tumor dissemination, not all the procedures are necessary and performed, usually necessitating one to three of the different peritonectomy procedures.

8.5. Hypertermic Intraperitoneal Chemotherapy (HIPEC)

After having made complete surgical cytoreduction with an absent or minimal residual disease (less than 2.5 mm tumor diameter), some catheters are inserted into the abdominal cavity and a perfusion of saline solution is made. Usually, depending on patient BMI, the quantity of saline solution perfused in the abdomen may vary between 2 and 6 l. After reaching a determined temperature, antiblastic drugs are perfused. The most frequently used antiblastic drugs include Mytomycin, Cisplatin, Oxaliplatin, Doxorubicin, and Taxol, which are chosen case by case depending on the origin of peritoneal carcinomatosis.

The peritoneal perfusion may lasts 30-90 minutes and it can be performed in condition of closed abdomen or open abdomen (coliseum technique) or a compromise between the two, with an abdominal wall small entrance suitable for the handling by the operator.

Hyperthermic perfusion can be obtained by heating the perfusion medium with a heat exchanger connected to the perfusion pump. The peritoneal cavity temperature considered optimal in terms of antitumor activity and antiblastic tumor tissue diffusion is 41.5-42.5 °C [23? , 24]. It is of absolute importance to control the temperature of organs and bowels during the procedure. Excessive temperature of intraperitoneal tissue, more than 43 °C, is strongly correlated with lesions of the bowel wall and perforation, and also with necrosis of nerves, bladder or vases. To prevent excessive intraperitoneal temperature multiple temperature probes are placed within the peritoneal cavity to monitor the temperature. At the end of the procedure the perfused medium is removed from the peritoneal cavity.

8.6. Outcomes of CRS and HIPEC in gynecologic malignancies

Among patients affected by ovarian cancer, the performance CRS and HIPEC has been recognized to correlate with better overall and disease-free survival. Two recently published systematic reviews, which analyzed almost all the available international literature, concluded that this comprehensive treatment modality is a viable option in the management of patients with advanced stage III-IV disease, with potential benefits comparable with the current standard of care (conventional secondary cytoreduction or systemic chemotherapy) [15, 25]. In particular, median overall survival for primary and recurrent disease extrapolated from the studies reviewed ranged from 22 to 64 months with a median disease-free survival from 10 to 87 months [25]. Most of the studies among those reviewed showed that patients with complete CRS had the greatest benefit, with a 5-year survival rate ranging from 12 to 66% [15, 25].

About uterine cancer, indeed, there is very poor data about the outcome after CRS and HIPEC. However, a recent study on thirteen patients demonstrated a significant survival time in selected patients, suggesting in the future a more extensive role of this procedure in women with peritoneal carcinomatosis of endometrial origin [16]

9. Conclusive summary

Radical hysterectomy is still an important surgical procedure in gynecologic oncology. New technologies are changing hysterectomy techniques and integrated treatments (e.g., cytoreduction associated with HIPEC) could expand the surgical indications in gynecologic oncology.

Despite the benefits of the minimally invasive (laparoscopic or robotic surgery) radical hysterectomy its adoption has been slow in cancer treatment [1]. In fact, both laparoscopic and robotic approaches showed favorable mobility profiles in comparison to open techniques. However, some issues have likely contributed to the slow adoption of these techniques. In general these cancer treatments are technically demanding procedures and the relatively uncommon diagnosis of cervical cancer have probably slowed the adoption of these techniques. Another issue is the cost of introducing robotic surgery in a gynecologic operative theater. Furthermore, data about oncologic long term outcomes of minimally invasive surgery are relatively sparse [1].

Acknowledgments

The authors would like to thank the whole collaborating staff of the Westfälische Wilhelms-Universität Münster (WWU), Universitât dal Friûl, and IRCCS CRO of Aviano.

In particular, we would like to thank Alexandra Woltering. In addition, we are also grateful to Prof. Diego Marchesoni and Dr Lorenza Driul for their help and suggestions.

Author details

Ambrogio P Londero[1]*, Serena Bertozzi[2], Luca Martella[2], Giulio Bertola[2], Giorgio Giorda[2], Angelo Calcagno[3], Arrigo Fruscalzo[4,5], Ralph J Lellé[4]

*Address all correspondence to: ambrogio.londero@gmail.com

1 Unit of Obstetrics and Gynecology, S. Polo Hopsital, Monfalcone (GO), Italy

2 IRCCS CRO, Aviano (PN), Italy

3 Clinic of Obstetrics and Gynecology, University of Udine, Italy

4 Clinic of Obstetrics and Gynecology, University of Münster, Germany

5 Unit of Obstetrics and Gynecology, St. Franziskus-Hospital, Münster, Germany

References

[1] Wright JD, Herzog TJ, Neugut AI, Burke WM, Lu YS, Lewin SN, et al. Comparative effectiveness of minimally invasive and abdominal radical hysterectomy for cervical cancer. Gynecol Oncol. 2012;**127**:11–17. .

[2] Kim HS, Kim TH, Suh DH, Kim SY, Kim MA, Jeong CW, et al. Success factors of laparoscopic nerve-sparing radical hysterectomy for preserving bladder function in patients with cervical cancer: a protocol-based prospective cohort study. Ann Surg Oncol. 2014;.

[3] Meigs JV. Removal of the pelvic lymph nodes in cancer of the uterine cervix; transperitoneal (taussig) and retroperitoneal (nathanson) dissection. Gynecol Prat. 1951; **2**:127–39.

[4] Lellé RJ, Heidenreich W, Lück HJ, Schneider J. Morley inter-iliac transverse incision in gynecologic operations. Geburtshilfe Frauenheilkd. 1995;**55**:695–698.

[5] Toussaint MN, Hillemanns HG. Graduated ruler for making a transverse suprapubic incision. J Gynecol Obstet Biol Reprod (Paris). 1989;**18**:99–101.

[6] Lellé RJ, Schneider J. Intentional incision of the urinary bladder during complex gynecologic oncologic operations. Zentralbl Gynakol. 1996;**118**:228–231.

[7] Roberts WH, Krishingner GL. Comparative study of human internal iliac artery based on Adachi classification. Anat Rec. 1967;**158**:191–196. .

[8] Querleu D, Morrow CP. Classification of radical hysterectomy. Lancet Oncol. 2008; **9**:297–303. .

[9] Patsner B. Closed-suction drainage versus no drainage following radical abdominal hysterectomy with pelvic lymphadenectomy for stage IB cervical cancer. Gynecol Oncol. 1995;**57**:232–234. .

[10] Choi CH, Lee JW, Lee YY, Kim HJ, Song T, Kim MK, et al. Comparison of laparoscopic-assisted radical vaginal hysterectomy and laparoscopic radical hysterectomy in the treatment of cervical cancer. Ann Surg Oncol. 2012;**19**:3839–3848. .

[11] Ditto A, Martinelli F, Bogani G, Gasparri ML, Di Donato V, Zanaboni F, et al. Implementation of laparoscopic approach for type B radical hysterectomy: a comparison with open surgical operations. Eur J Surg Oncol. 2015;**41**:34–39. .

[12] Al-Shammaa HAH, Li Y, Yonemura Y. Current status and future strategies of cytoreductive surgery plus intraperitoneal hyperthermic chemotherapy for peritoneal carcinomatosis. World J Gastroenterol. 2008;**14**:1159–1166.

[13] Glehen O, Schreiber V, Cotte E, Sayag-Beaujard AC, Osinsky D, Freyer G, et al. Cytoreductive surgery and intraperitoneal chemohyperthermia for peritoneal carcinomatosis arising from gastric cancer. Arch Surg. 2004;**139**:20–26. .

[14] Chua TC, Yan TD, Saxena A, Morris DL. Should the treatment of peritoneal carcinomatosis by cytoreductive surgery and hyperthermic intraperitoneal chemotherapy still be regarded as a highly morbid procedure?: a systematic review of morbidity and mortality. Ann Surg. 2009;**249**:900–907. .

[15] Chua TC, Robertson G, Liauw W, Farrell R, Yan TD, Morris DL. Intraoperative hyperthermic intraperitoneal chemotherapy after cytoreductive surgery in ovarian cancer peritoneal carcinomatosis: systematic review of current results. J Cancer Res Clin Oncol. 2009;**135**:1637–1645. .

[16] Delotte J, Desantis M, Frigenza M, Quaranta D, Bongain A, Benchimol D, et al. Cytoreductive surgery with hyperthermic intraperitoneal chemotherapy for the treatment of endometrial cancer with peritoneal carcinomatosis. Eur J Obstet Gynecol Reprod Biol. 2014;**172**:111–114. .

[17] Bakrin N, Cotte E, Sayag-Beaujard A, Raudrant D, Isaac S, Mohamed F, et al. Cytoreductive surgery with hyperthermic intraperitoneal chemotherapy for the treatment of recurrent endometrial carcinoma confined to the peritoneal cavity. Int J Gynecol Cancer. 2010;**20**:809–814.

[18] Bristow RE, del Carmen MG, Pannu HK, Cohade C, Zahurak ML, Fishman EK, et al. Clinically occult recurrent ovarian cancer: patient selection for secondary cytoreductive surgery using combined PET/CT. Gynecol Oncol. 2003;**90**:519–528.

[19] Bharwani N, Reznek RH, Rockall AG. Ovarian cancer management: the role of imaging and diagnostic challenges. Eur J Radiol. 2011;**78**:41–51. .

[20] Pasqual EM, Bertozzi S, Bacchetti S, Londero AP, Basso SMM, Santeufemia DA, et al. Preoperative assessment of peritoneal carcinomatosis in patients

undergoing hyperthermic intraperitoneal chemotherapy following cytoreductive surgery. Anticancer Res. 2014;**34**:2363–2368.

[21] Sugarbaker PH. Peritonectomy procedures. Ann Surg. 1995;**221**:29–42.

[22] Gilly FN, Carry PY, Sayag AC, Brachet A, Panteix G, Salle B, et al. Regional chemotherapy (with mitomycin C) and intra-operative hyperthermia for digestive cancers with peritoneal carcinomatosis. Hepatogastroenterology. 1994;**41**:124–129.

[23] Sugarbaker PH, Chang D. Results of treatment of 385 patients with peritoneal surface spread of appendiceal malignancy. Ann Surg Oncol. 1999;**6**:727–731.

[24] Sugarbaker PH. Observations concerning cancer spread within the peritoneal cavity and concepts supporting an ordered pathophysiology. In Sugarbaker PH. (ed.) Peritoneal carcinomatosis: principles of management. Springer US; 1996. p79–100.

[25] Bijelic L, Jonson A, Sugarbaker PH. Systematic review of cytoreductive surgery and heated intraoperative intraperitoneal chemotherapy for treatment of peritoneal carcinomatosis in primary and recurrent ovarian cancer. Ann Oncol. 2007;**18**:1943–1950.

Chapter 7

Pelvic Exenteration for the Management of Pelvic Malignancies

Daniel Paramythiotis, Konstantinia Kofina and Antonios Michalopoulos

Additional information is available at the end of the chapter

http://dx.doi.org/10.5772/61083

Abstract

Pelvic exenteration is a surgical procedure first described by Brunschwig in 1948 as a curative or palliative treatment for pelvic and perineal tumors. It is actually a radical operation, involving en bloc resection of pelvic organs, including reproductive structures, bladder, and rectosigmoid. In patients with recurrent cervical and vaginal malignancy, it is associated with a 5-year survival of more than 50%. In spite of advances in surgical management, consequences such as stomas, are still frequently unavoidable for radical tumor excision. Most candidates for this procedure have been diagnosed with recurrent cervical cancer that has previously been treated with surgery and radiation, or radiation alone. Complications of pelvic exenteration are more severe than those of standard resection of a colorectal carcinoma, so it is not commonly performed, including wound infection, wound dehiscence (also described as burst abdomen) the creation of fistulae (perineal-fecal, uretero-vaginal, between conduit and perineal wound), urinary tract infections, perineal hernias and intestinal obstruction. Patients need to be carefully selected and counseled about risks and long-term issues related to the surgery. A comprehensive evaluation is required in order to exclude unresectable or metastatic disease. Evolution of the technique through laparoscopy and minimally invasive surgery may result in a reduction of morbidity and mortality.

Keywords: Pelvic exenteration, gynecologic cancer

1. Introduction

Pelvic exenteration was first described by Brunschwig and his colleagues of New York's Memorial Hospital in 1948 [1] and was initially performed as a palliative surgical intervention

INTECH
open science | open minds

© 2015 The Author(s). Licensee InTech. This chapter is distributed under the terms of the Creative Commons Attribution License (http://creativecommons.org/licenses/by/3.0), which permits unrestricted use, distribution, and reproduction in any medium, provided the original work is properly cited.

for extended recurrences of gynecologic carcinomas. These tumors usually invade local tissues, such as the urinary tract and the rectum, the pelvic sidewall, and the urogenital diaphragm. Thus, an en bloc removal of the lower abdomen structures and reconstruction procedures to preserve urinary, intestinal, and sexual functions was taken into consideration.

Since Brunschwig's time, the improvement of surgical techniques (such as stapling devices, separate urinary conduits, and pelvic reconstruction), postoperative critical care units, antibiotic and thromboembolic prophylaxis, and the wisest selection of patients, have improved the morbidity and mortality rates associated with the procedure. The survival rates range from 16–60% for recurrent cervical cancer for 5 years postoperatively, 40% for uterine cancer with variations depending on the histology of the tumor, and 62% for vulvar cancer (according to Forner and Lampe's study). The postoperative survival is up to 8 months, and surgical mortality rate reaches about 23% [2].

Due to this improvement, the procedure has gained widespread acceptance in selective centers, even though it presents a negative mutilating impact [3]. A thorough preoperative examination must be performed in order to select those patients to whom the operation is appropriate. The recurrence should be confirmed by its clinical symptoms and biopsy results and a complete laboratory evaluation and a thorough imaging study (C.T., M.R.I, bone scan) must be performed to evaluate the patient's health status and the presence of metastases.

Pelvic exenteration is, therefore, a procedure that can be performed either for a tumor concerning general surgery (rectal cancer) or obstetrics (female reproductive system tumors).

2. Classification

Pelvic exenteration is actually a radical operation, involving an en bloc resection of pelvic organs, including reproductive structures, bladder, rectosigmoid, and sacrum. The patient undergoing pelvic exenteration is, usually, placed in the lithotomy position, and, through a midline incision, all the organs of the abdomen and pelvis are thoroughly explored.

Pelvic exenterations can be classified into three groups:

- **Anterior** pelvic exenteration

It involves the resection of central pelvic organs, bladder, and distal ureters bilaterally, but spares the gastrointestinal tract. The rectosigmoid, anus, and lower portion of the posterior vagina are left intact.

- **Posterior** pelvic exenteration

The procedure removes the central organs together with the rectosigmoid, but spares the anterior vagina, urinary bladder, and ureters.

- **Total** pelvic exenteration

This form is actually the combination of the previous types. It involves the evacuation of all pelvic organs, including the bladder, rectum, vagina, urethra, vulva, clitoris and anus [2]. It

http://dx.doi.org/10.5772/61083

requires the creation of a urinary conduit for urine (continent or non-continent), a colostomy, as well as the reconstruction of the pelvic floor and vagina using flaps, such as the rectus abdominus or gracilis muscles [4].

- Other than those common forms, new types have been introduced, as **extended** exenterations, which include abdominosacral resection, and **individualized** approaches.

This original classification of pelvic exenteration addresses only the nature of the pelvic viscera removed. Some authors have suggested a new sub-classification that takes the levator ani muscle as a reference point and offers a better definition of the extent of resection and the anatomical changes associated with each operation [5]: supra-levator (Type I), infra-levator (Type II), combined with vulvectomy (Type III).

It is expected that not every case fits in one of the above-mentioned specific types of the procedure, therefore the technique should be be individualized (Fig. 1).

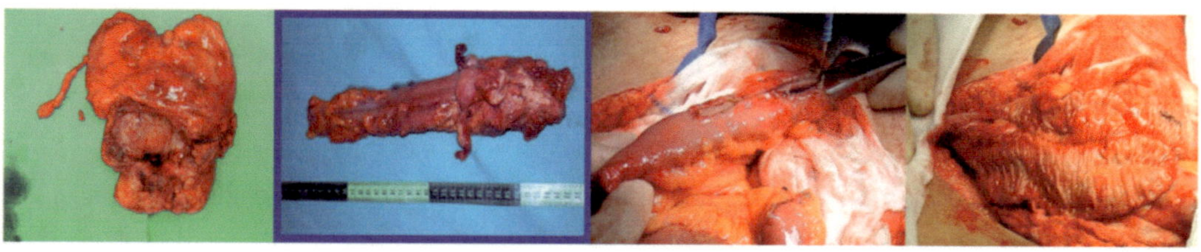

Figure 1. Total pelvic exenteration in a female patient in which bladder, rectum-sigmoid, and vagina were resected and needed a small intestine neocyst for urinary conduit.

In most patients, resection of the rectosigmoid with low primary re-anastomosis is not advisable in the irradiated pelvis, and, thus, total exenteration should be preferred. Efforts to preserve either the bladder (anterior exenteration) or rectosigmoid may evoke severe postoperative complications and often malfunction of the preserved organs; such efforts may not be advisable in some cases [6]. Anterior and total supra-levator pelvic exenteration in patients with gynecological malignancies is feasible with orthotopic reconstruction of the lower urinary tract [7].

Depending on the classification type, the procedure may include end-sigmoid colostomy or low rectal anastomosis, continent or noncontinent urinary diversion, and vaginal and pelvic reconstruction [8]. Moreover, such procedures may also be combined with intra-operative radiation therapy for improved disease control at the pelvic sidewall or possible cancer positive margins.

3. Indications

The most common indication for exenteration is cervical carcinoma that is advanced or has recurred after radiotherapy (about 70%), followed by locally advanced rectal carcinoma (about

10%) in both men and women. In these cases, it is a feasible surgical procedure, especially in selected medical centers and in selected patients with tumors of size less than 30 mm, negative surgical margins, and no lymph node involvement [9].

As postoperative complications remain high, operative procedures and their indications must be continuously revised to further reduce the complication rate in the selected cases. An international register of exenterations should be organized in order to generate prospective data on different aspects of this procedure. These oncologic data would give therapists the opportunity to advise patients and to define the indications and contraindications of this operation more precisely.

4. Contraindications

Pelvic exenteration is not feasible in all cases of gynecologic and rectal cancers. Contraindications to exenteration include incurability indications such as distant metastases, invasion of pelvic bones and major blood vessels, pelvic wall musculature involvement, and intraperitoneal disease [10].

Advanced age should not be considered as a contraindication to a potentially curable case, as in some series it is shown that duration of surgery, blood loss, length of hospital stay, and complication rates do not increase with age [11]. However, other factors such as high level BMI, hypertension, or pulmonary disease may influence the outcome [12].

On the other hand, there are considerable differences concerning indications and contraindications, preoperative staging, and adjuvant therapy for pelvic exenteration between each study [13]. Therefore, further studies are needed to specify these factors for each gynecologic tumor.

Although pelvic exenteration can be performed in cases of recurrent rectal cancer without distant metastases, several studies have demonstrated that negative surgical margin status (R0 excision) is the most important prognostic factor for disease-free survival. Recurrent disease, preoperative BMI greater than 30 and lymphatic invasion are considered as poor prognostic factors. Therefore, invasion through the greater sciatic notch, metastasis to the para-aortic lymph nodes, extensive pelvic sidewall involvement, tumor encasement of the iliac vessels, lower limb oedema, ASA IV-V and probably invasion into S1 or S2 are contraindications for the operation.

5. Complications

Most complications after pelvic exenteration are considered to be caused by a compromised healing of the irradiated tissues [14] and are classified in many categories by many studies [15, 16, 17] with a different rate of occurrence.

Early complications include, among others, pyelonephritis, venous thrombosis, lesion of the obturator nerve, abscess, partial necrosis of the gracilis flap, and chronic obstructive pulmonary disease decompensation. Late complications are fistulas (colon-skin, bladder-vagina, ileum-vagina), pyelonephritis, and incisional hernia. Ileo-ileal anastomosis failure, colostomy obstruction, pelvic peritonitis, septic shock, seroma of the lower limb, and pelvic lymphedema, when they occur, are considered as major complications.

Cooperation with general surgeons and/or urologists, intensive postoperative management, and patient selection are crucial in order to reduce the complication rates and improve the patients' survival.

6. Outcome and prognosis

The median time of recurrence, after initial treatment, is 18–24 months and occurs in 20%–30% of patients initially treated with concomitant chemotherapy for recurrent cervical cancer [18]. The overall limitation of the existing studies is the heterogeneity in the inclusion criteria and the consideration of several types of cancers (of the cervix, endometrium, vulva, and ovaries) [19]. A 5-year survival of 46% for primary advanced and 17% for locally recurrent rectal cancer has also been shown [20].

Factors that influence prognosis after pelvic exenteration are feasibility of complete microscopic and macroscopic resection (R0), lymph node involvement, lymph vascular invasion, perineural invasion, tumor grade, size of recurrence, pelvic sidewall involvement, interval between primary treatment and pelvic exenteration, total number of tumor-invaded organs, mesorectum lymph node involvement, and vascular emboli on pretherapeutic biopsies [21].

A resection with sound margins, histologically confirmed, is both mandatory and very often possible in selected cases after pelvic exenteration (85%). Patients treated with total microscopic and macroscopic resection have a 5-year overall survival of 53%, and this percentage is even higher in patients without lymph node metastases [21], so the resection margins are a significant factor for the determination of the patient's survival. Patients, whose margins were negative, had longer survival than those with positive margins. Surgical margin status is an important predictive factor for the recurrence of the disease, as well. There are several techniques in order to achieve total microscopic and macroscopic resection. R0 microscopic resection has better survival rates than total macroscopic ones, where part of the tumor is left behind, as shown microscopically. Therefore, it is accepted extending into wider planes to ensure that radical excision is achieved [22].

Many patients with locally recurrent colorectal cancer are precluded from postoperative radiation because of previous radiation's limitations or proximity to radiosensitive pelvic organs; therefore, an alternative is intraoperative radiation therapy (IORT). Complications such as delayed healing, wound breakdown, ureteric stenosis, peripheral neuropathy, and osteonecrosis can occur after this combination of treatments. Radiation therapy at the time of pelvic exenteration doesn't change survival and recurrence outcomes for cervical, vaginal, or vulvar cancer. However, patients with clinical indications for intraoperative radiation therapy at the time of pelvic exenteration have worse prognosis compared to those who do not require this procedure. The surgeon may consider performing a laterally extended endo-pelvic resection to decrease local recurrence or consider palliative treatment options [23].

7. Quality of life

Although patients report gastrointestinal symptoms and a decline in physical function after pelvic exenteration, most adjust well, returning to almost baseline functioning within a year. Patients should be counseled that many symptoms are likely to improve in the first postoperative months, as they adapt to their changed health status [24]. The systematic assessment of quality of life, sexuality, and body self-image by standardized questionnaires should be incorporated into the evaluation of the surgical outcome of such radical procedures [25].

Surgery is always a life-changing action, impacting physical, psychosocial, and sexual functions, as well as body image [26]. As part of preoperative counseling and postoperative support, the changes, especially in a woman's body image following pelvic exenteration, must be taken into consideration. Some patients report improved quality of life following surgery, with decreased narcotic requirements and malodorous discharge. Most women, however, note a decline in sexual quality of life (almost diminished), whereas body image, physical ability, and social functions are all decreased. The available data suggest that deficits in sexuality, attractiveness, and self-confidence are significantly higher postoperatively compared to preoperatively [27]. These changes are more obvious in younger patients and those who do not undergo vaginal reconstruction. However, overall function, and mental and emotional quality of life are comparable to those preoperatively and patients may report similar levels of emotional well-being and general quality of life when compared to healthy women.

During the last fifteen years, reconstructive surgery has significantly improved with a benefit on the quality of life of women. Reconstructive techniques should be carefully individualized after an adequate counseling about expectations and risks [28]. Soft-tissue reconstructions are needed to reduce complications, to secure the pelvic floor, and to reconstruct the vagina in selected patients. Commonly used flaps for perineal and vaginal reconstruction include the gracilis myocutaneous, vertical rectus abdominis myocutaneous (VRAM), and posterior thigh flaps. Thus, a muscle and fascia–sparing flap based on the deep inferior epigastric perforator artery (DIEP) seems to be a promising flap for this kind of reconstruction and could replace the transverse rectus abdominis myocutaneous pedicled (TRAM) flap, according to a study that showed a decrease in donor-site abdominal morbidity when using the DIEP flap compared with the TRAM flap [29]. The transverse musculocutaneous gracilis (TMG) flap can also be used for reconstructions after total pelvic exenteration. It does not lead to functional deficits, complicate the abdominal stomas, or weaken the abdominal wall. It reduces the length of operation and, moreover, donor defect and scars are minimal [30, 31].

In order to improve the quality of life, many techniques of continent urinary diversion have also been developed during the last decades. Such techniques improve continent mechanisms, and decrease postoperative complications and surgical difficulty (using the Studer or the Indiana technique). Today, the most popular forms of continent urinary diversions used in gynecology oncology are Mainz pouch, Indiana pouch, and Miami pouch. There are no differences in postoperative complications between patients with continent and no-continent conduits except that stone formation may be more common in patients with continent conduits [32]. Many advances of these techniques have been made, and physicians have learned to manage complications in a more conservative way [33, 34].

http://dx.doi.org/10.5772/61083

8. Conclusions

Management options for pelvic cancers include surgical resection and radiotherapy, hormonal therapy, cytotoxic chemotherapy, and targeted therapy with novel biological agents, or palliative measures . When a recurrence occurs, the tumor may be locally advanced but still limited to the pelvis; however, previous treatment with high doses of radiation makes surgical resection a difficult procedure with an increased rate of complications. There is no optimal treatment regimen. Rather, one must consider the patient's performance status and prior treatment history. Patients need to be carefully selected and counseled about risks and long-term issues related to pelvic exenteration.

Many questions regarding the indication for such radical operations, the handling of irradiated tissues, and the optimal reconstructive procedures are still open and demand multi-institutional controlled trials to be answered. Laparoscopic and minimally invasive surgery and application of this technology to radical pelvic surgery, including pelvic exenteration, are challenging and may result in a reduction of morbidity and mortality.

Pelvic exenteration needs surgical experience, specialized medical centers and an interdisciplinary team, and has become an intriguing operation for advanced central pelvic recurrence in patients with gynecologic, urinary, or rectal cancer that were previously treated with radiotherapy only. Further studies on the exenterative procedures for the management of such advanced pelvic malignancies are necessary.

Author details

Daniel Paramythiotis*, Konstantinia Kofina and Antonios Michalopoulos

*Address all correspondence to: danosprx@med.auth.gr

1st Propedeutic Surgical Clinic, A.H.E.P.A. University Hospital, Aristotle University of Thessaloniki, Greece

References

[1] Brunschwig A. Complete excision of pelvic viscera for advanced carcinoma; a one-stage abdominoperineal operation with end colostomy and bilateral ureteral implantation into the colon above the colostomy. Cancer 1948; 1(2): 177-183.

[2] Diver EJ, Rauh-Hain A, del Carmen MG. Total pelvic exenteration for gynecologic malignancies. Int J Surg Oncol 2012;2012:693535.

[3] Bacalbasa N, Balescu I. Pelvic exenteration – reconsidering the procedure. J Med Life 2015; 8(2):146-149.

[4] Mayer Hope J, Pothuri B. The role of palliative surgery in gynecologic cancer cases. Oncologist 2013; 18: 73-79.

[5] Gadducci A, Tana R, Cosio S, Cionini L. Treatment options in recurrent cervical cancer (Review). Oncol Lett 2010; 1(1): 3-11.

[6] Dreyer G, Snymn LC, Mouton A, Lindeque BG. Management of recurrent cervical cancer. Best Practice & Research Clinical Obstetrics and Gynaecology. 2005; 19(4): 631-644.

[7] Ungar L, Palfalvi L, Novak Z. Pelvic exenteration without external urinary or fecal diversion in gynecological cancer patients. Int J Gynecol Cancer 2006; 16: 364-368.

[8] de la Garza J, Wilson SS, Behbakht K. Total pelvic exenteration with a split-thickness skin graft neovagina, continent orthotopic neobladder and rectal reanastomosis, resulting in no eternal ostomies and adequate sexual function. Gynecol Oncol 2009; 115: 312-313.

[9] Hockel M, Dornhofer N. Pelvic exenteration for gynaecological tumours: achievements and unanswered questions. Lancet Oncol 2006; 7: 837-847.

[10] Mayer Hope J, Pothuri B. The role of palliative surgery in gynecologic cancer cases. Oncologist 2013; 18: 73-79.

[11] Huang M, Iglesias DA, Westin SN, et al. Pelvic exenteration: impact of age on surgical and oncologic outcomes. Gynecol Oncol 2014; 132(1): 114-118.

[12] Kaur M, Joniau S, D'Hoore A, Vergote I. Indications, techniques and outcomes for pelvic exenteration in gynecological malignancy. Curr Opin Oncol 2014; 26(5): 514-520.

[13] Marnitz S, Dowdy S, Lanowska M, et al. Exenterations 60 years after first description. Results of a survey among US and German gynecologic oncology centers. Int J Gynecol Cancer 2009; 19: 974-977.

[14] Petruzziello A, Kondo W, Hatscback SB, et al. Surgical results of pelvic exenteration in the treatment of gynecologic cane. World J Surg Oncol 2014; 1: 279-285.

[15] Tanaka S, Nagase S, Kaiho-Sakuma M, et al. Clinical outcome of pelvic exenteration in patients with advanced or recurrent uterine cervical carcinoma. Int J Clin Oncol 2014; 19: 133-138.

[16] Goldberg GL, Sukumvanich P, Einstein MH, et al. Total pelvic exenteration: The Albert Einstein College of Medicine/Montefiore Medical Center experience (1987 to 2003). Gynecol Oncol 2006; 101: 261-268.

[17] Jager L, Nilsson PJ, Radestad AF. Pelvic exenteration for recurrent gynecologic malignancy. A study of 28 consecutive patients at a single institution. Int J Gynecol Cancer 2013; 23: 755-762.

[18] Peiretti M, Zapardiel I, Zanagnolo V, et al. Management of recurrent cervical cancer: a review of the literature. Surg Oncol 2012; 21: 59-66.

[19] Sardain H, Lavoue V, Laviolle B, et al. Prognostic factors for curative pelvic exenterations in patients with recurrent uterine cervical or vaginal cancer. Int J Gynecol Cancer 2014; 24: 1679-1685.

[20] Nielsen MB, Rasmussen PC, Lindegaard JC, Laurberg S. A 10-year experience of total pelvic exenteration for primary advanced and locally recurrent rectal cancer based on a prospective database. Colorectal Dis 2012; 14(9): 1076-1083.

[21] Chiantera V, Rossi M, De Iaco P, et al. Pelvic exenteration of recurrent endometrial adenocarcinoma. A retrospective multi-institutional study about 21 patients. Int J Gynecol Cancer 2014; 24: 880-884.

[22] Warren OR, Solomon MJ. R0 resection, not surgical technique, is the key consideration in pelvic exenteration surgery. Tech Coloproctol 2015; 19(2): 117-118.

[23] Backes FJ, Billingsley CC, Martin DD, et al. Does intra-operative radiation at the time of pelvic exenteration improve survival for patients with recurrent, previously irradiated cervical, vaginal, or vulvar cancer? Gynecol Oncol 2014; 135: 95-99.

[24] Rezk YA, Hurley KE, Carter J, et al. A prospective study of quality of life in patients undergoing pelvic exenteration: Interim results. Gynecol Oncol 2013; 128(2): 191-197.

[25] Fotopoulou C, Neumann U, Kraetschell R, et al. Long-term clinical outcome of pelvic exentertion in patients with advanced gynecologic malignancies. J Surg Oncol 2010; 101: 507-512.

[26] Westin S, Rallapalli V, Fellman B, et al. Overall survival after pelvic exenteration for gynecologic malignancy. Gynecol Oncol 2014; 134: 546-551.

[27] Kaur M, Joniau S, D'Hoore A, et al. Pelvic exenteration for gynecological malignancies. A study of 36 cases. Int J Gynecol Cancer 2013; 22: 889-896.

[28] Chiantera V, Rossi M, De Iaco P, et al. Morbidity after pelvic exenteration for gynecological malignancies. A retrospective multicentric study of 230 patients. Int J Gynecol Cancer 2014; 24: 156-164.

[29] Huffman LB, Randolph LK, McCann GA, et al. Options for repair of rectus abdominis myocutaneous perineal/vaginal flap prolapse: A case series. Gynecol Oncol Rep 2014; 7: 1-3.

[30] Qiu SS, Jurado M, Hontanilla B. Comparison of TRAM versus DIEP flap in total vaginal reconstruction after pelvic exenteration. Plast Reconstr Surg 2013; 132(6): 1020-1027.

[31] Kaartinen IS, Vuento MH, Hyoty MK, et al. Reconstruction of the pelvic floor and the vagina after total pelvic exenteration using the transverse musculocutaneous gracilis flap. J Plast Rec & Aesthetic Surg 2015; 68: 93-97.

[32] Urh A, Soliman PT, Schmeler K, et al. Postoperative outcomes after continent versus incontinent urinary diversion at the time of pelvic exenteration for gynecologic malignancies. Gynecol Oncol 2013; 129(3): 580-585.

[33] Panici PB, Angioli R, Plotti F, et al. Continent ileocolonic urinry diversion (Rome pouch) for gynecologic malignancies: technique and feasibility. Gynecol Oncol 2007; 107: 194-199.

[34] Bradford LS, Rauh-Hain JA, Schorge J, et al. Advances in the management of recurrent endometrial cancer. Am J Clin Oncol 2015; 38(2): 206-212.

Section 5

B-Lynch Compression Suture as an Alternative to Peripartum Hysterectomy

Chapter 8

B-Lynch Compression Suture as an Alternative to Paripartum Hysterectomy

Christopher Balogun-Lynch and Tahira Aziz Javaid

Additional information is available at the end of the chapter

http://dx.doi.org/10.5772/61295

Abstract

Obstetrics haemorrhage is a major killer of women of all categories of class, religion, social and economic status. Women of third world countries suffer the most adversity because of poor resources and infrastructure. In major substandard care, haemorrhage emerges as the major cause of severe maternal morbidity in almost all 'near miss' audits in both developed and developing countries [1, 2, 24].

Paripartum Haemorrhage (PPH) is a serious medical problem. There are about 14 million case occurrences worldwide each year, with a fatality rate of 1%. A total of 140,000 women die each year [3]. Hysterectomy has a very damaging effect in a woman's life. In some ethnic communities this can cause marital breakdown and psychological problems. Hysterectomy for PPH needs experts who have technical skills as usually the patients are already in a compromised condition. Ninety percent of the reason for PPH is because of uterine atony.

Keywords: Pph blynch suture, Hysterectomy, Balloon tamponade, Pph teaching

1. Introduction

1.1. The Management of paripartum haemorrhage: Avoiding paripartum hysterectomy

1.1.1. Medical management

The medical management of PPH includes using ecbolic such as syntometrin, carboprost, and misoprostol. Sometimes medical management fails and it becomes necessary to proceed to surgical treatment to save the woman's life.

INTECH
open science | open minds

© 2015 The Author(s). Licensee InTech. This chapter is distributed under the terms of the Creative Commons Attribution License (http://creativecommons.org/licenses/by/3.0), which permits unrestricted use, distribution, and reproduction in any medium, provided the original work is properly cited.

1.2. Conservative surgical management

1.2.1. Bimanual compression of the uterus

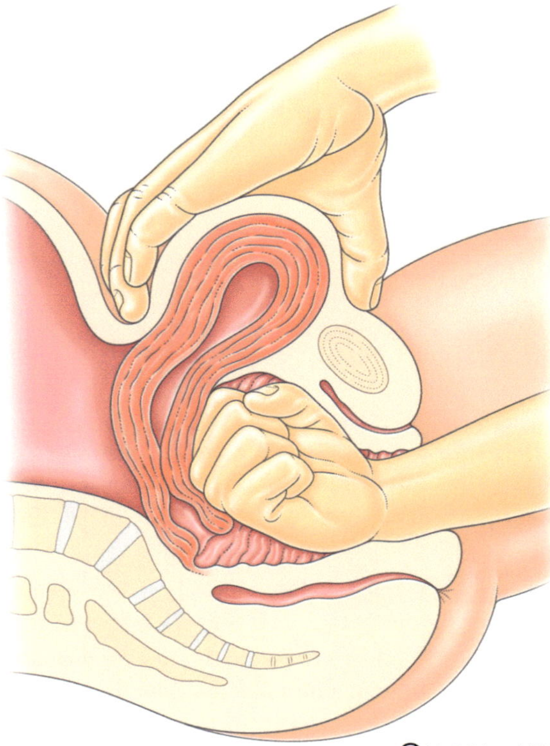

Figure 1. The fist of one hand is placed deep into the vagina while the other hand firmly compresses the uterine fundus in an effort to control bleeding.

1.2.2. Balloon tamponade

- **Bakri Balloon**
- **Sengstaken-Blakemore Oesophageal Catheter**
- **Rusch Balloon**

Balloon Tamponade was invented to simulate the old traditional way of intrauterine compression by packing and creating intrauterine uniform tension to reduce infection risk. Various balloons have been tried and tested, but we choose to discuss the common varieties [4-6, 8, 9]. The Scottish Confidential Audit of Severe Maternal Morbidity identified 64 cases where balloon tamponade was used for the management of major PPH; hysterectomy was averted in 50 (78%) of the women [10].

Bakri Balloon

In PPH following vaginal delivery, a balloon, such as Bakri, with sufficient volume capacity can be inserted into the uterine cavity after excluding any retained products and also ascertaining that there is no genital tract trauma. The volume of fluid depends on what is needed to achieve haemostasis. The capacity of the balloon is important to correlate with the tension that must be created to maintain adequate haemostasis. This is the tamponade test [11, 12]. The duration of tamponade will vary with the efficiency of bleeding control. Before its complete removal, the balloon could be deflated but left in place to ensure that bleeding does not re-occur.

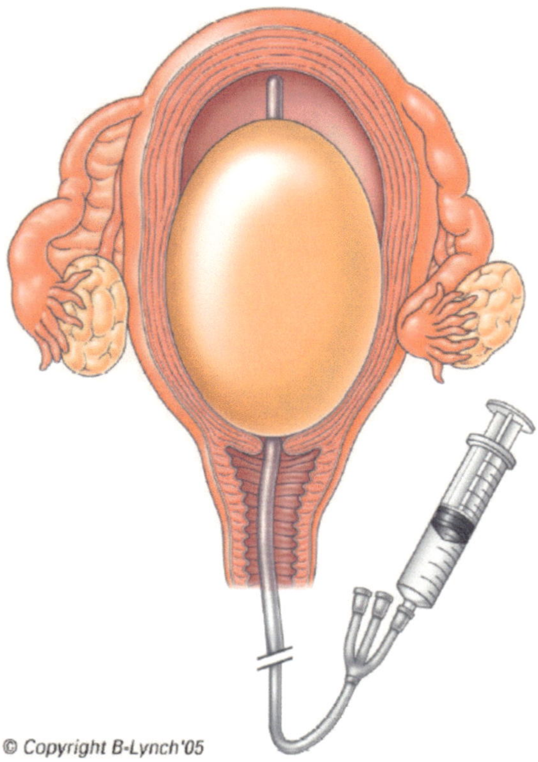

Sengstaken-Blakemore Oesophageal Catheter

Originally used to control gastro-oesophageal bleeding (haematemesis). If there is continued PPH following balloon tamponade, there becomes an urgent need for laparotomy to arrest haemorrhage.

1.2.3. Haemostatic compression suture

A review published in 2005 of 32 cases of B-Lynch suture reported success in all but one case [13]. In 2002, Hayman et al. described a modified compression suture that does not require

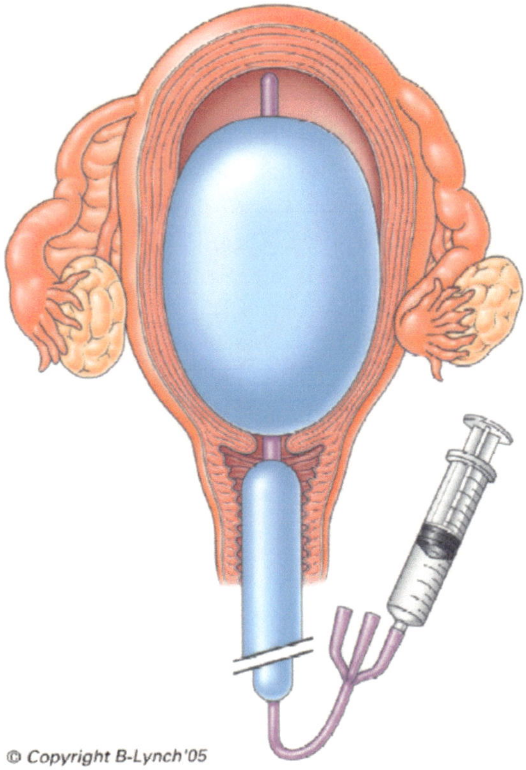

hysterotomy [14] and in 2007, Ghezzi et al. reported success in 10 of 11 cases of women managed with this modified technique [15-17].

It has been reported that hysterectomy was averted in 42 of 52 cases (81%) women where haemostatic brace suturing was used for the management of major PPH [10, 14].

The physiological effect of compression suture is twofold:

- **First is to enhance the effect of the uterine muscle to slide into contraction**
- **Secondly, it occludes the vascular spaces within the uterus**

Since the b-lynch compression suture was first described by B-Lynch et al. (1997), evidence suggest that over 8,000 women lives and uteri have been saved (B-Lynch personal Communication 2014, www.cblynch.co.uk) [17].

- **Hayman technique**

The potential disadvantages are:

- Restricted drainage of endometrium because anterior and posterior surfaces are compressed
- Suture anchoring causes shouldering, therefore when it slips can cause venous return occlusion, central ischemia, and there is a possibility of pyometra of the uterus

http://dx.doi.org/10.5772/61295

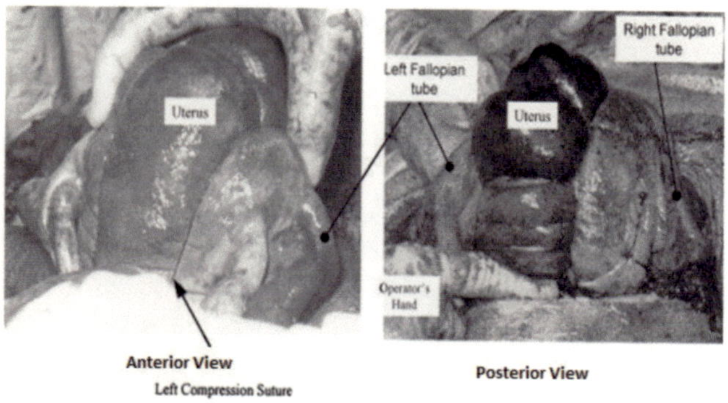

- **Homeostatic multiple square suture method**

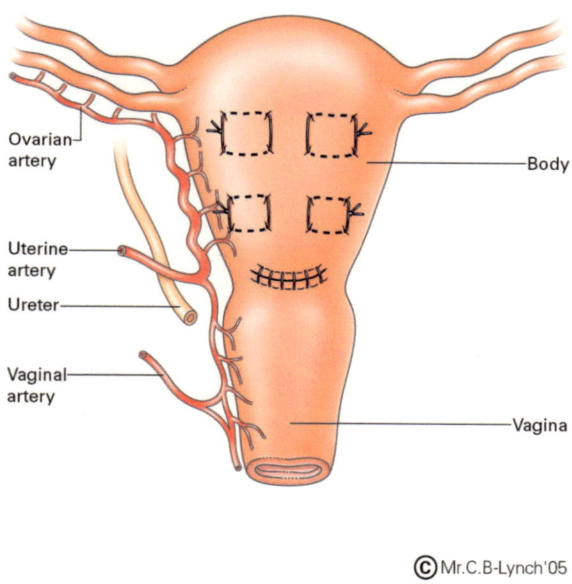

Special Features

- It pierces the uterus 32 times.
- It impairs involution. It causes poor drainage because the cavity is occluded.
- It does not close all transverse branches of the vascular supply.
- It can cause pyometra and Asherman Syndrome [18].
- It is difficult to apply and to achieve haemostasis when there is DIC (Disseminated Intravascular coagulation).

- **The B-Lynch suture compression suture avoiding paripartum hysterectomy**

Indications

- Uterine atony
- Polyhydroamnios
- Multiple pregnancy
- Big baby
- Eclampsia
- Uterine anomaly
- Abruptio placentae
- Abnormal placentation

Requirements for B-Lynch suture are as follows:

- Lloyd Davis or frog-legged position essential
- The uterus must be exteriorised
- Basic surgical competence required
- Bi-manual compression to test for potential success
- Transverse lower segment incision should be made
- Uterine cavity checked, explored, and evacuated
- A 70-mm half circle guarded needle (code: w3709) mounted on a 90-cm monocryl No. 1 (Ethicon, Somerville, N.J.) or Catgut suture is appropriate
- Apply suture correctly with even tension (no shouldering)
- Allow free drainage of blood, debris, and inflammatory material.
- Check bleeding control vaginally, using swabs and instruments

B-Lynch suture illustration of technique

In vitro illustration of the B-Lynch suture application

In vivo illustration of properly applied B-Lynch suture

The special features of B-Lynch suture are:

- Even tension
- Free drainage of cavity
- No shouldering
- Facilitates involution

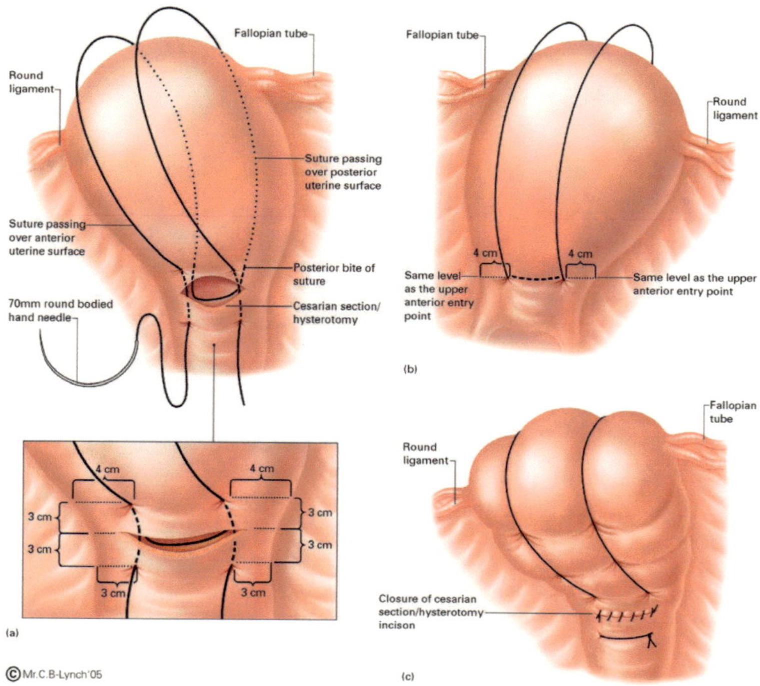

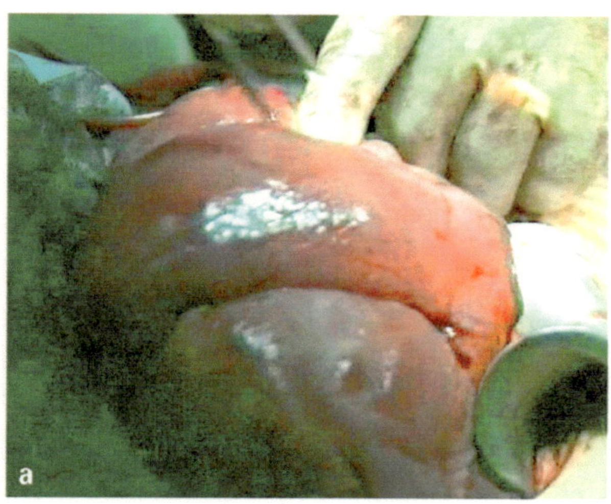

Figure 2. Anterior View

- Easy to confirm haemostasis
- Confirms no retained products and uterine cavity is empty
- Easy to confirm no decidual tear/trauma

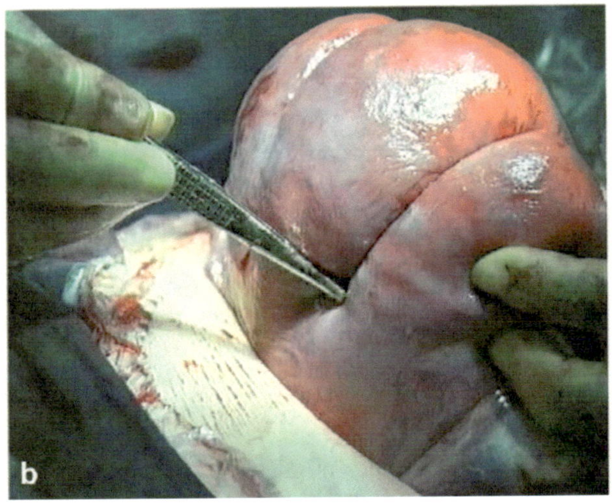

Figure 3. Posterior View

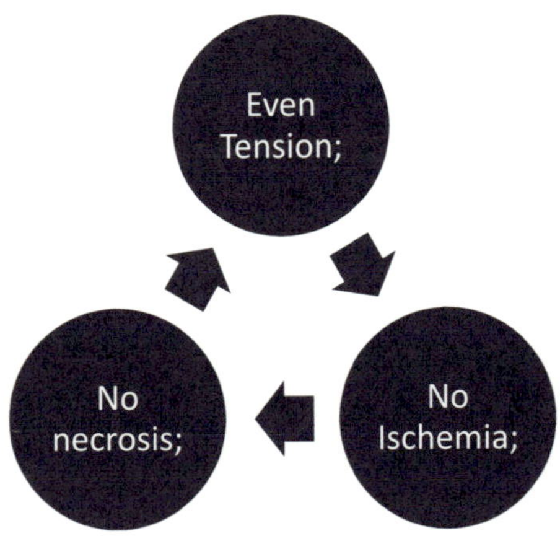

- The uterus should be exteriorised and the surgeon demonstrates to his assistant bimanual compression and ante version. The second assistant checks the vagina to ensure that bleeding is controlled and the surgical technique will work.

Causes of failure

- Placenta percreta
- Wrong technique causing uterine necrosis
- Uncontrolled DIC
- No pre-operative test done
- Not properly applied

• Delayed application

1.2.4. Other surgical techniques

• **Internal iliac artery ligation**

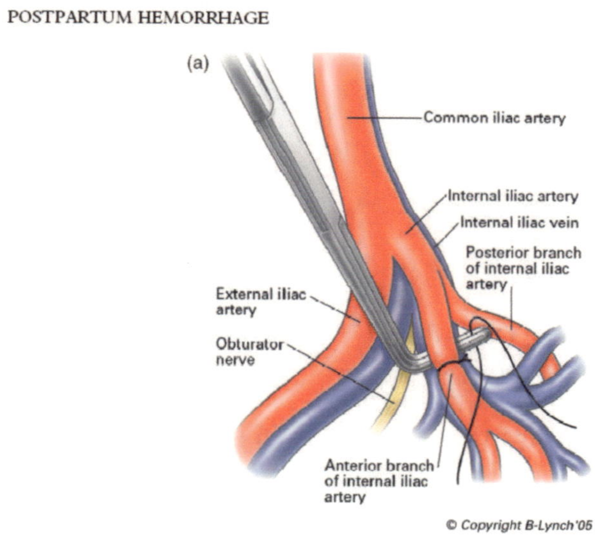

A recent case series describes 84 women with PPH from various causes who underwent internal iliac artery ligation as the first-line surgical intervention. Hysterectomy was required in 33 (39%) of the women.

• **Stepwise de vascularisation (sites of vascular occlusion)**

This is relatively easy to perform but time consuming.

• **Selective arterial occlusion or embolisation by interventional radiologist**

A 2002 review summarised a case series totalling 100 women and reporting 97% success with selective arterial embolisation for obstetric haemorrhage [19, 20].

Method	No. of Cases	Success Rate
B-Lynch + other compression sutures	94	90.4 %
Arterial embolization	218	91.0 %
Arterial ligation	264	83.7 %
Uterine balloon tamponade	135	83.7 %

Table 1. Table of success rate of each procedure (B-Lynch Personal Communication 2014)

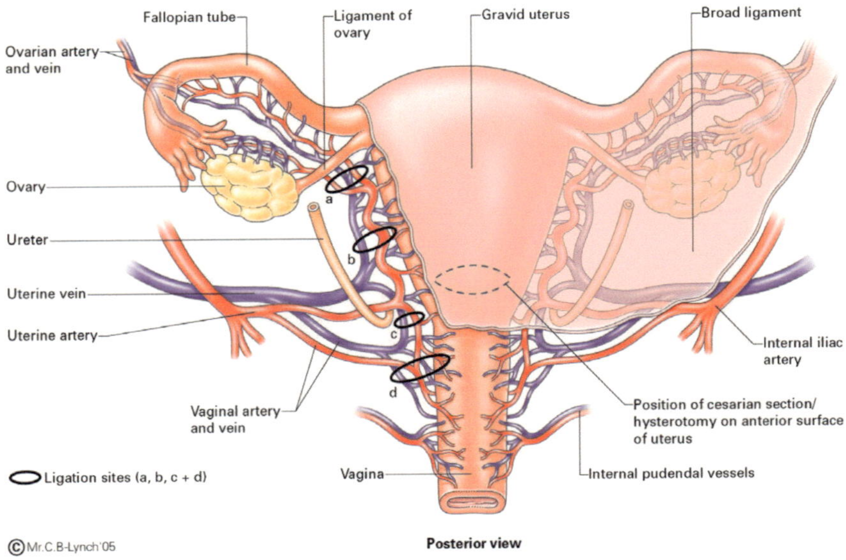

1.3. Learning to treat paripartum haemorrhage: A spectrum of modern teaching/learning modalities

William Osler (1849-1919) brought forth the concept of bedside teaching/learning in the 19th century [21]. Although more than a century has passed since he first aired this concept, and the practice of medicine both at the bedside and in the office has changed radically, his statement remains entirely true with regard to the management of PPH.

Specifically, in recent years training in emergency obstetric skills (including PPH training) has moved from the traditional clinical teaching, normally conducted in the labour ward to specific, targeted skills and scenario-based courses that utilise mannequins and simulators most often away from the bedside. Such changes are currently seen as necessary, largely as a result of the limitations of traditional clinical teaching when it comes to genuine patient encounters in an emergency situation [22].

The authors are grateful to Professor Amr El Noury of Cairo University for designing the poster that provides a stepwise guide to the management of PPH (Figure 12).

2. The drivers for paripartum haemorrhage training

The incidence of PPH is increasing in both developed and developing countries [23, 24]. The World Health Organization (WHO) has set a goal to reduce maternal mortality by 75% by 2015, mainly by reducing maternal deaths related to PPH by training health workers in both developing and developed countries [25]. Recently, further initiatives have been undertaken by WHO in addressing women's health crisis in Africa by providing a report on women's health in the African Region [26].

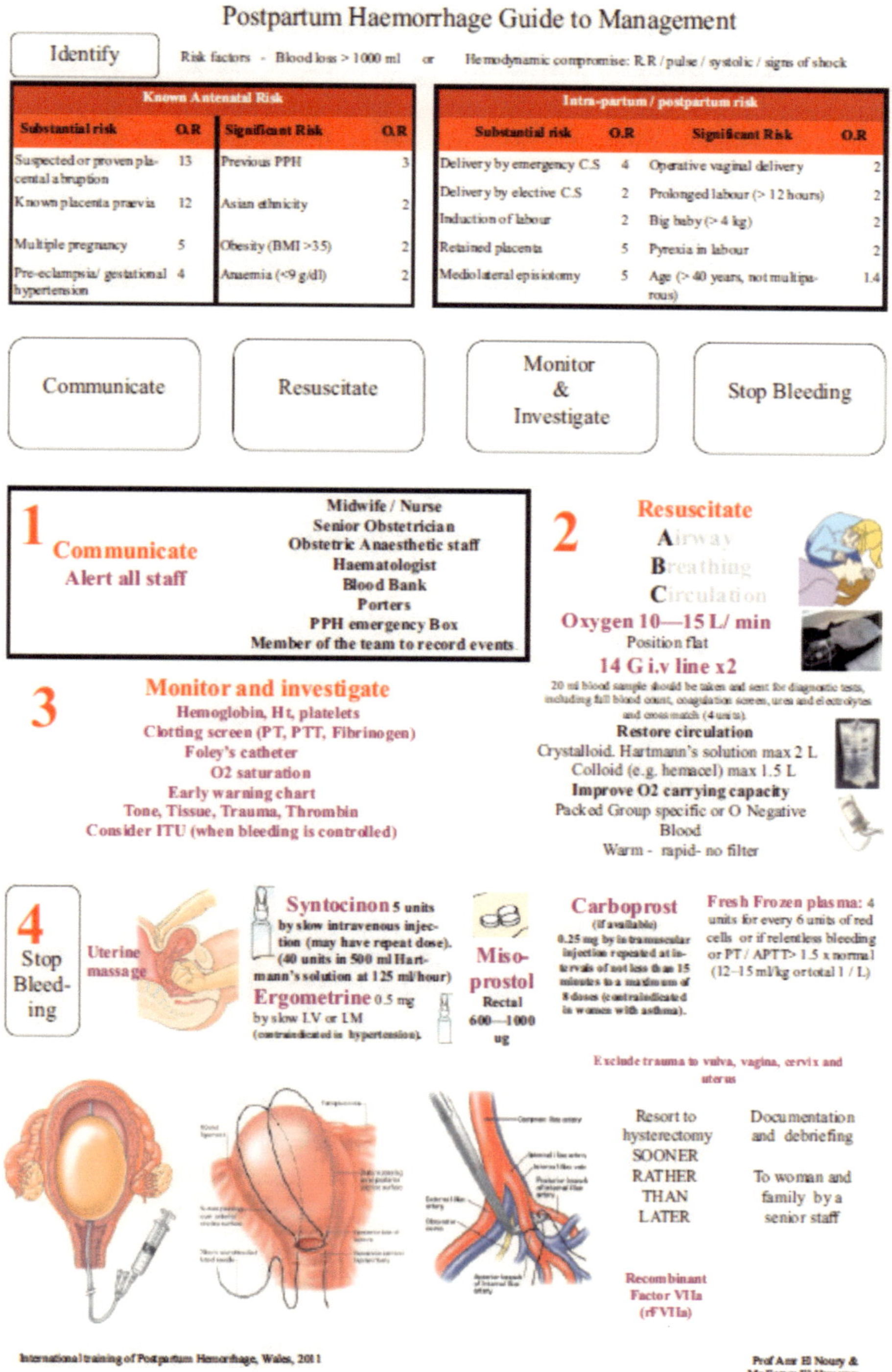
Postpartum Haemorrhage Guide to Management
Identify
Risk factors - Blood loss > 1000 ml or Hemodynamic compromise: R.R / pulse / systolic / signs of shock
Known Antenatal Risk
Substantial risk O.R
Suspected or proven placental abruption 13
Known placenta praevia 12
Multiple pregnancy 5
Pre-eclampsia/ gestational hypertension 4
Significant Risk O.R
Previous PPH 3
Asian ethnicity 2
Obesity (BMI >35) 2
Anaemia (<9 g/dl) 2
Intra-partum / postpartum risk
Substantial risk O.R
Delivery by emergency C.S 4
Delivery by elective C.S 2
Induction of labour 2
Retained placenta 5
Mediolateral episiotomy 5
Significant Risk O.R
Operative vaginal delivery 2
Prolonged labour (> 12 hours) 2
Big baby (> 4 kg) 2
Pyrexia in labour 2
Age (> 40 years, not multiparous) 1.4
Communicate
Resuscitate
Monitor & Investigate
Stop Bleeding
1 Communicate
Alert all staff
Midwife / Nurse
Senior Obstetrician
Obstetric Anaesthetic staff
Haematologist
Blood Bank
Porters
PPH emergency Box
Member of the team to record events
2 Resuscitate
Airway
Breathing
Circulation
Oxygen 10—15 L/ min
Position flat
14 G i.v line x2
Restore circulation
Crystalloid. Hartmann's solution max 2 L
Colloid (e.g. hemacel) max 1.5 L
Improve O2 carrying capacity
Packed Group specific or O Negative Blood
Warm - rapid- no filter
3 Monitor and investigate
Hemoglobin, Ht, platelets
Clotting screen (PT, PTT, Fibrinogen)
Foley's catheter
O2 saturation
Early warning chart
Tone, Tissue, Trauma, Thrombin
Consider ITU (when bleeding is controlled)
4 Stop Bleeding
Uterine massage
Syntocinon 5 units by slow intravenous injection (may have repeat dose). (40 units in 500 ml Hartmann's solution at 125 ml/hour)
Ergometrine 0.5 mg by slow I.V or I.M (contraindicated in hypertension).
Misoprostol Rectal 600—1000 ug
Carboprost (if available)
Fresh Frozen plasma: 4 units for every 6 units of red cells or if relentless bleeding or PT / APTT> 1.5 x normal (12–15 ml/kg or total 1 / L)
Exclude trauma to vulva, vagina, cervix and uterus
Resort to hysterectomy SOONER RATHER THAN LATER
Documentation and debriefing
To woman and family by a senior staff
Recombinant Factor VIIa (rFVIIa)
International training of Postpartum Hemorrhage, Wales, 2011
Prof Amr El Noury & Mr Essam El Hamamy

Figure 4. [31].

Prior to these efforts, the Federation of Gynaecology and Obstetrics (FIGO), together with the Confederation of Midwives (ICM), advocated the Global Initiative on the Prevention of Postpartum Haemorrhage in 2004. In addition, both organizations recommend that every skilled attendant (doctors, nurses, and midwives) likely to be present at birth have training in uterine massage and bimanual compression. The same document also advises that all skilled birth attendants have access to technical training in administering uterotonics and other techniques such as intravenous infusions and tamponade balloons, and that every doctor who can perform laparotomy be provided with surgical training to perform 'simple conservative surgery' for PPH including compression sutures and sequential devascularisation [27].

In the UK, successive Confidential Enquiries into Maternal Deaths have linked the increased numbers of deaths from PPH to recent changes in medical training. Specifically, the reduction in the overall length of obstetric training and in working hours during training may have reduced the amount of experience gained compared with the experiences obtainable in the past. Moreover, these reports have shown a trend towards sub-specialization among consultants in the UK, and those with a special interest in obstetrics do not necessarily have highly developed surgical skills. These reports recommend regular 'fire drills' or 'skills drills' for the modern management of PPH for all grades of staff in every obstetric unit.

The 2004 and 2007 Confidential Enquiry into Maternal and Child Health (CEMACH) reports repeatedly highlight the role of inadequate clinical care, as well as poor communication and teamwork, within labour ward teams and suggest that as many as half of all maternal deaths might be prevented with better care [28, 29]. Following this line of thought, the 2011 CEMACH report recommended that all units should have protocols in place for the identification and management of PPH and that all clinicians responsible for the care of pregnant women, antenatal, postnatal, and intrapartum, including those practicing in the community, should carry out regular skills training for such scenarios [30]. The need for such a recommendation follows the 2007 survey among obstetric trainees in London that documented a reported decline in the numbers of individuals who could manage major PPH. 44.6% of respondents felt confident to perform a caesarean hysterectomy, whereas a similar number (41.7%) could apply a B-Lynch suture, and a much smaller number (27.1%) could dissect the ureter if need be. Additionally, a few respondents were less confident in performing any surgical procedure necessary in the management of major obstetric haemorrhage. This finding may have serious implications in the provision of out of hours senior cover for maternity units in the future (32).

The Scottish Confidential Audit of Severe Maternal Morbidity 2008 highlighted errors and substandard care in the management of women who have sustained PPH. It is essential that blood transfusion service and laboratory test results are obtained and not ignored. There should be teamwork and efficient equipment to comply with PPH management. Any deficiency could be improved with adequate and target training.

The UK Obstetric Surveillance System (UKOSS) publication [34] echoes the growing recognition articulated that prompt action is essential in managing PPH. Those who provide care should try to do so within the first 2 hours of the diagnosis and certainly not beyond a delay of 6 hours. Morbidity rises sharply after 2 hours, when it becomes much more likely that hysterectomy will be necessary.

3. Modalities of training: Hands-on training

Hands-on training is a simple method for an on-the-job facilitator who works with small numbers of participants to teach them certain procedural applications. The working concept is to prepare the trainee at a workstation to mimic the procedure or scenario, let them practice it, and then review their competency.

This model of training is suitable for teaching practical skills such as the application of bimanual compression of the uterus, the uterine brace suture, uterine tamponade, etc. However, because of the small number of participants, it is not suitable to teach communication skills.

4. Lecture-based training

PPH is one of the catastrophic events where proper management requires a variety of hospital workers with different unique expertise. It is often difficult to get all these people together to arrange a simulation or hands-on training, and lecture-based teaching may be more appropriate. All staff should attend, obstetric physicians, midwives, nurses, house staff, anaesthesia providers, scrub technicians, and unit secretaries participate in the same formal classroom instruction. The purpose is for all team members to hear the same material, to learn the same teamwork language and behaviours, and to feel empowered to flatten hierarchy. The participants from varying disciplines should be allowed ample opportunity for conversation and sharing of varying points of view. It is mandatory that the team should be able to understand each other's roles and competing interests that may not be self-evident.

5. Simulation

There are two types of simulators, those with high and low fidelities. The high fidelity type is often used to describe computer driven simulators, whereas the term low fidelity is used to describe simulators that are not computer controlled. High fidelity is desirable in simulation, because the more contextually accurate is the simulation-based instruction, the more likely the learning that takes place will transfer to the reality of applied practice. The disadvantages of this type of training include costs, the need to remove clinicians from clinical care, and a lack of realism compared with the clinicians' own experience [35, 36].

Simulation-based training is an appropriate proactive approach for reducing errors and risk in obstetrics, improving teamwork and communication, and giving students a multiplicity of transferable skills to improve their performances. The drivers for simulation include patient safety, limitation of current educational processes, shortening of the training period, high risk emergencies, and the pressure of health care agencies in an attempt to reduce malpractice concerns [37, 38, 39]. Haemorrhage drills and simulation-based training may help providers achieve timely and coordinated responses [40]. Protocols may help to standardise management in cases of PPH, thereby minimizing unnecessary errors or delays in care [41].

Only a few models have been used for PPH training. Deering et al. used a standard obstetric birthing model equipped with an inflatable uterus to simulate uterine atony. The residents were assessed upon completion of this exercise. The authors found that the majority were unable to correct the haemorrhage within 5 minutes and half made at least one error, either in the dose or the route of administration of medications used to arrest the bleeding [41, 42].

Teamwork training in a simulation setting resulted in improvement of knowledge, practical skills, communication, and team performance in acute obstetric situations. Training in a simulation centre did not further improve outcome compared with training in a local hospital [40].

A simple low fidelity model has been used for the past few years by the authors. It is made of knitted wool and has an incision-like opening in the lower part to give the impression of a Paripartum uterus after the baby and the placenta have been expelled, along with the blood supply of the uterus and the ovaries. It is a useful tool to learn the placement of a B-Lynch or other type of compression suture and it also gives one the ability to practice a form of step-wise devascularisation.

6. Invaluable resources for PPH training

1. For PPH hands-on training and workshops, visit http://www.pphinternationaltraining.org/.
2. A short video demonstration of the B-Lynch suturing technique. This video is presented in real video format. There is a link provided to download, which is available at: http://www.cblynch.co.uk/video-of-an-operation-demonstrating-the-b-lynch-suturing-technique/.
3. Internet-based training. Visit The Global Library on Women's Medicine, launched November 2008 and is available at: www.glowm.com.
4. Poster of the B-Lynch suture technique to be displayed in the labour ward. This is available at: www.sapienspublishing.com/pph_pdf/PPH_ Poster.pdf.
5. Pocket manual of the synopsis of PPH. A special leaflet or wall chart summarising the immediate action that needs to be taken when PPH occurs. www.sapienspublishing.com/pph_pdf/PPH- Guidelines.pdf.
6. A Comprehensive Textbook of Paripartum Haemorrhage, 1st edition, 2006, edited by B-Lynch (43). This first standalone textbook describes a comprehensive guide to evaluation, management, and surgical intervention for PPH. Available at: www.sapienspublishing.com and also from www.glowm.com.
7. PPH issue of Best Practice & Research Clinical Obstetrics & Gynaecology [44].

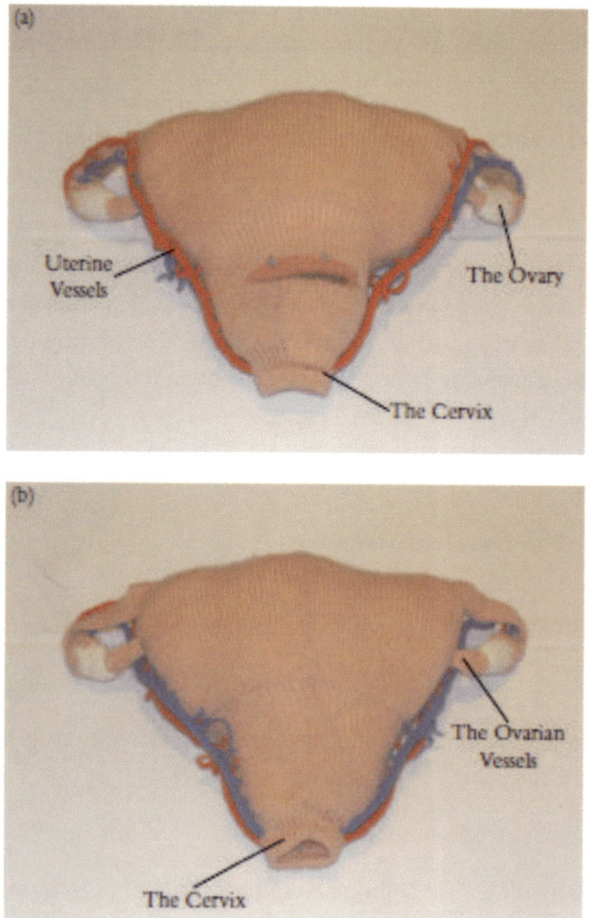

Figure 5. Uterine model (a) front view and (b) rear view.

7. Courses and workshops

A number of workshops that provide PPH training have been developed. These are available as either separate or part of other obstetric emergencies such as Advanced Life Support in Obstetrics (ALSO) [45], Maternal Obstetrics Emergency Trauma (MOET) [46] and Practical Obstetric Multi Professional Training (PROMPT) course [47]. The International Training and Workshop for the Management of Massive PPH Group was set up in 2009 in London with the objective to provide hands-on training and workshops in the management of PPH. The group is chaired by the senior author and includes experts who are renowned for their expertise in the management of PPH across the world.

The International Training Group has organized and run regular courses in Milton Keynes and South Wales, UK, all of which were very successful. Recently, the group has run a series of study days and workshops in both Cairo and Alexandria with successful feedback response. It seems that this training program and workshop would be beneficial to other developing countries to reduce maternal mortality rate from PPH [48].

Simulators should be put together to give the candidate and trainees the confidence of feeling a real life situation.

Multiple training modalities are used to accomplish knowledge transfer for modern management of PPH. All are necessary, as it is clear that the traditional methods of reading or attending a lecture are insufficient to prepare the trainee for responsible action when it is needed in an emergency situation. Like many other skills in medicine, the training necessary to attend to a patient who has a life-threatening haemorrhage cannot be thought of as 'see one, do one, and teach one'.

8. Essentials for effective training

- Regular drills and skills training are essential in the management of PPH.
- Trainees should be allowed dedicated and protected time for training.
- Simulation of obstetric procedures and emergencies can only augment, not replace, the learning that occurs by caring for actual patients.
- In-house training is cheap and associated with improved outcomes.
- Funding should be available for training to reduce the cost of medical litigation as a result of substandard care.
- Team work is essential for proper coordination of the management.
- Above all, patients and their relatives must be kept fully informed at all stages of management.

9. Post-operative care

9.1. Intensive and high-dependency unit

Once the bleeding has been controlled and initial resuscitation has been completed, continuous close observations in either intensive care unit or high-dependency unit is required. The recording of the observation on an obstetric early-warning score system would help in the early identification of continuous bleeding, especially in cases that are not apparent, as recommended by CEMACH [2].

http://dx.doi.org/10.5772/61295

10. Debriefing

To avoid future complications and need of care, an action plan should be prepared for all subsequent pregnancy management.

11. Conclusion

B-Lynch suture has been the most effective and successful haemostatic compression suture to prevent maternal morbidity and mortality by controlling severe PPH and in reducing the need for hysterectomy. It is important that conservative methods such as bi-manual compression of the uterus, balloon tamponade, and, more recently, endometrial suction and selective arterial occlusion are carried out before hysterectomy is considered.

Author details

Christopher Balogun-Lynch[1*] and Tahira Aziz Javaid[2]

*Address all correspondence to: Christopherbl@aol.com

1 Milton Keynes General Hospital, Oxford Deanery, UK

2 Wexham Park Hospital, Slough, UK

References

[1] Confidential Enquiry into Maternal and Child Health. Why Mothers Die 2000-2002. Sixth Report on Confidential Enquiries into Maternal Deaths in the United Kingdom. London: RCOG Press; 2004 [www.cemach.org.uk/Publications/ Saving-Mothers-Lives-Report-2000-2002.aspx].

[2] Confidential Enquiry into Maternal and Child Health. Saving Mothers Lives 2003-2005. Seventh Report on Confidential Enquiries into Maternal Deaths in the United Kingdom. London: CEMACH; 2006 [www.cemach.org.uk/getattachment/ 927cf18a-735a-47a0-9200-cdea103781c7/Saving-Mothers--Lives- 2003-2005_full.aspx].

[3] Estimates developed by WHO, UNICEF, and UNFPA. Maternal mortality in 2000. Geneva: Department of Reproductive Health and Research, World Health Organization; 2004.

[4] Ikechebelu JI, Obi RA, Joe-Ikechebelu NN. The control of paripartum haemorrhage with intrauterine Foley catheter. J Obstet Gynecol. 2005; 25:70-2.

[5] Bakri YN, Amri A, Abdul Jabbar F. Tamponade-balloon for obstetrical bleeding. Int J Gynaecology Obstet. 2001;74:139-42.

[6] Chan C, Rizvi K, Tham KF, Arulkumaran S. The use of a Sengstaken-Blakemore tube to control paripartum haemorrhage. Int J Obstet Gynecol. 1997;58:251-2.

[7] Condous GS, Arulkumaran S, Symonds I, Chapman R, Sinha A, Razvi K. The 'tamponade test' in the management of massive paripartum haemorrhage. Obstet Gynecol. 2003;101:767-72.

[8] Akhter S, Begum MR, Kabir Z, Rashid M, Laila TR, Zabeen F. Use of a condom to control massive paripartum haemorrhage. Medscape General Medicine. 2003;5:38.

[9] Keriakos R, Mukhopadhyay A.The use of the Rusch balloon for management of severe paripartum haemorrhage. J Obstet Gynecol. 2006;26:335-8. (10) RCOG Guideline no 52, Paragraph 6.5.3.

[10] Penney G, Brace V. Near miss audit in obstetrics. Curr Opin Obstet Gynecol. 2007;19:145-50.

[11] Frenzel D, Condous GS, Papageorghiou AT, McWhinney NA. The use of the 'tamponade test' to stop massive obstetric haemorrhage in placenta accreta. BJOG. 2005;112:676-7.

[12] B-Lynch C, Coker A, Lawal AH, Abu J, Cowen MJ. The B-Lynch surgical technique for the control of massive paripartum haemorrhage: An alternative to hysterectomy? Five cases reported. BJOG 1997;104:372-5.13. (www.cblynch.com/HTML/bjog1.html) (B-Lynch et al, 1997).

[13] Harma M, Gungen N, Ozturk A. B-Lynch uterine compression suture for paripartum haemorrhage due to placenta praevia accreta. Aust N Z J Obstet Gynaecol. 2005;45:93-5.

[14] Hayman RG, Arulkumaran S, Steer PJ. Uterine compression sutures: Surgical management of PPH. Obstet Gynecol. 2002;99:502-6.

[15] Ghezzi F, Cromi A, Uccella S, Raio L, Bolis P, Surbek D. The Hayman technique: A simple method to treat paripartum haemorrhage. BJOG. 2007;114:362-5.

[16] Hwu YM, Chen CP, Chen HS, Su TH. Parallel vertical compression sutures: a technique to control bleeding from placenta praevia or accreta during caesarean section. BJOG. 2005;112:1420-3.

[17] Kafali H, Demir N, Soylemez F,Yurtseven S. Hemostatic cervical suturing technique for management of uncontrollable paripartum haemorrhage originating from the cervical canal. Eur J Obstet Gynecol Reprod Biol. 2003;110:35-8. (20) (B-Lynch personal Communication 2014).

[18] Ochoa et al. ObGy 99:506-509, Obstet Gynecol. 2000 Jul;96(1):129-131.

[19] Salomon LJ, deTayrac R, Castaigne-Meary V, Audibert F, Musset D, Ciorascu R, et al. Fertility and pregnancy outcome following pelvic arterial embolization for severe post-partum haemorrhage. A cohort study. Hum Reprod. 2003;18:849-52.

[20] Descargues G, Mauger Tinlot F, Douvrin F, Clavier E, Lemoine JP, Marpeau L. Menses, fertility, and pregnancy after arterial embolization for the control of paripartum haemorrhage. Hum Reprod. 2004;19:339-43.

[21] McCall N, ed. The Portrait Collection of Johns Hopkins Medicine: A Catalog of Paintings and Photographs at The Johns Hopkins University School of Medicine and The Johns Hopkins Hospital. Baltimore: The Johns Hopkins University School of Medicine, 1993.

[22] To WW. Training in emergency obstetric skills: Is it evidence-based? Hong Kong Med J 2011;17:141-6.

[23] Knight M, Callaghan WM, Berg C, et al. Trends in postpartum haemorrhage in high resource countries: A review and recommendations from the international paripartum haemorrhage collaborative group. BMC Pregnancy Childbirth. 2009;9:55.

[24] Karoshi M, Keith L. Challenges in managing PPH in resource-poor countries. Clin Obstet Gynecol. 2009;52:285-98.

[25] World Health Organization. Guidelines for the Management of Paripartum Haemorrhage and Retained Placenta. Geneva: World Health Organization, 2009.

[26] World Health Organization. Addressing the Challenge of Women's Health in Africa. Report of the Commission on Women's Health in the African Region. Brazzaville, Republic of Congo: WHO, 2011.

[27] International Federation of Obstetrics and Gynaecology. International Confederation of Midwives. International Joint Policy Statement. FIGO/ICM global initiative to prevent post-partum haemorrhage. J Obstet Gynaecol Can. 2004;26: 1100-2.

[28] Confidential Enquiry into Maternal and Child Health (CEMACH). Why Mothers Die: Report on Confidential Enquiries into Maternal Deaths in the United Kingdom 2002-2004 Triennial Report. London: RCOG Press, 2004: 94-103.

[29] Confidential Enquiry into Maternal and Child Health. Saving Mothers' Lives. The Seventh Report of the Confidential Enquiries into Maternal Deaths in the United Kingdom, 2005-2007 Triennial Report. London: RCOG, 2007:78-85.

[30] Cantwell R, Clutton-Brock T, Cooper G, et al. Saving Mothers' Lives: Reviewing maternal deaths to make motherhood safer: 2006-08. The Eighth Report on Confidential Enquiries into Maternal Deaths in the United Kingdom. BJOG. 2011;118 (Suppl. 1): 71-776.

[31] B-Lynch et al. Text book of PPH 2nd Edition Sapien Pubishing.

[32] Ghaem-Maghami S, Brockbank E, Bridges J. Survey of surgical experience during training in obstetrics and gynaecology in the UK. J Obstet Gynaecol. 2006;26:297-301.

[33] Lennox C, Marr L. Scottish Confidential Audit of Severe Maternal Morbidity 2008: 6th Annual Report. Edinburgh: NHS Quality Improvement Scotland, 2010.

[34] Kayem G, Kurinczuk JJ, Zarko A, et al. Obstetric Surveillance System (UKOSS), uterine compression sutures for the management of severe PPH. Obstet Gynecol. 2011;117:14-20.

[35] Gardner R, Raemer DB. Simulation in obstetrics and gynaecology. Obstet Gynecol Clin North Am. 2008;35:97-127.

[36] Fuchs KM, Miller RS, Berkowitz RL. Optimizing outcomes through protocols, multidisciplinary drills, and simulation, Semin Perinatol. 2009;33:104-8 39.

[37] Clark EA, Fisher JR, Arafeh J, Druzin M. Team training/simulation. Clin Obstet Gynecol. 2010;53:265-77.

[38] Andreatta PB, Bullough AS, Marzano D. Simulation and team training, clinical obstetrics and gynaecology. Clin Obstet Gynecol. 2010;53:532-44.

[39] Skupski DW, Lowenwirt IP, Weinbaum FI, et al. Improving hospital systems for the care of women with major obstetric haemorrhage. Obstet Gynecol. 2006;107:977-83.

[40] Rizvi F, Mackey R, Barrett T, McKenna P, Geary M. Successful reduction of massive paripartum haemorrhage by use of guidelines and staff education. BJOG. 2004;111:495-8.

[41] Merién AE, Van de Ven BW. Multidisciplinary team training in a simulation setting for acute obstetric emergencies: A systematic review. Obstet Gynecol. 2010;115:1021-31.

[42] Ennen CS, Satin AJ. Training and assessment in obstetrics: The role of simulation. Best Pract Res Clin Obstet Gynaecol. 2010;24:747-58.

[43] B-Lynch et al. Text book of PPH 2nd Edition Sapien Publishing.

[44] Deering SH, Chinn M, Hoddor J, et al. The use of a postpartum simulator for instruction and evaluation of residents. J Grad Med Educ. 2009;1:260-3.

[45] Alfirevic Z, ed. Paripartum haemorrhage. Best Pract Res Clin Obstet Gynaecol. 2010;22:997-1170.

[46] Advanced life support in obstetrics (ALSO). http://www. also.org.uk/.

[47] Maternal Obstetrics Emergency Trauma (MOET). http://www.alsg.org/en/?q=moet

[48] Practical Obstetric Multi Professional Training (PROMPT). http://www.prompt-course.org/.

Section 6

Peripartum Hysterectomy

Chapter 9

Peripartum Hysterectomy

Zouhair O. Amarin

Additional information is available at the end of the chapter

http://dx.doi.org/10.5772/60942

Abstract

Peripartum hysterectomy is uncommon in modern obstetrics. It is mostly performed as an emergency procedure to control life-threatening haemorrhage. Despite recent technical advances in medicine, it is associated with high rates of morbidity and mortality. Peripartum hysterectomy constitutes a life-saving procedure.

Keywords: Hysterectomy, Peripartum, Postpartum haemorrhage

1. Introduction

Peripartum hysterectomy can be defined as the removal of the corpus uteri alone or with the cervix at the time of a caesarean section or within the puerperium. The removal of the uterus at caesarean section is referred to as caesarean hysterectomy, while the removal after vaginal birth is called postpartum hysterectomy. The operation may be performed as an emergency or as a planned procedure [1,2].

Although uncommon in modern obstetrics, peripartum hysterectomy is one of the most devastating complications in obstetrics. It represents a catastrophic end to a pregnancy to all women in general and to those wanting to maintain their fertility in particular [3,4].

Despite advances in medicine and surgery, peripartum hysterectomy is associated with high rates of morbidity, near miss and mortality. It is mostly performed as an emergency procedure to control torrential life-threatening haemorrhage and remains a life-saving procedure [1,2,5].

INTECH
open science | open minds

© 2015 The Author(s). Licensee InTech. This chapter is distributed under the terms of the Creative Commons Attribution License (http://creativecommons.org/licenses/by/3.0), which permits unrestricted use, distribution, and reproduction in any medium, provided the original work is properly cited.

2. History

Peripartum hysterectomy was proposed in 1768 by Joseph Cavallini in animal experiments. In 1823, James Blundell approved caesarean hysterectomy on a work based on rabbits. The first documented caesarean hysterectomy was performed by Horatio Storer in 1869. The patient died 68 h after surgery. In 1876, Eduardo Porro performed the first caesarean hysterectomy in which both the mother and baby survived. His patient was a 25-year-old primiparous dwarf. A constricting wire was passed around the cervix to control haemorrhage, and the uterus was excised. The abdominal wound was closed with silver wire. Various modifications followed, such as those of Godson in 1884 and Lawson in 1890 [6].

3. Incidence

In modern obstetrics, there are considerable differences in the incidence of emergency peripartum hysterectomy in different parts of the world, with higher figures in low-resource countries, while developed countries generally report lower rates [7,8]. The variations may be related to the standard of antenatal care, unbooked emergencies, obstetric care, differing rates of caesarean delivery, different patterns of parity, maternal age and the earlier recourse to hysterectomy due to the lack of adequate blood and blood banking facilities. In addition, certain conservative procedures involving interventional radiology may not be available in most developing countries [9].

In a recent review of relevant articles in English literature, the incidence of emergency peripartum hysterectomy ranged from 0.24 to 8.7 per 1000 deliveries [10].

4. Risk factors

Emergency peripartum hysterectomy was found to be more common following caesarean section than vaginal deliveries. In addition, there is a significant association between emergency peripartum hysterectomy and previous caesarean section and placenta praevia. The risk of emergency peripartum hysterectomy increases with the number of previous caesarean sections. There is an increased incidence of previous caesarean section in patients with placenta praevia and in patients with adherent placenta [11-23].

To estimate the magnitude of increased maternal morbidity associated with increasing number of caesarean deliveries, Silver et al. in a prospective observational cohort of 30,132 women who had caesarean delivery without labour in 19 academic centres over 4 years found that placenta accreta was present in 15 (0.24 %), 49 (0.31%), 36 (0.57 %), 31 (2.13 %), 6 (2.33 %) and 6 (6.74 %) women undergoing their first, second, third, fourth, fifth and sixth or more caesarean deliveries, respectively. Hysterectomy was required in 40 (0.65 %) first, 67 (0.42 %) second, 57 (0.90 %) third, 35 (2.41 %) fourth, 9 (3.49 %) fifth and 8 (8.99 %) sixth or more caesarean deliveries.

Furthermore, in women with praevia, the risk for placenta accreta was 3 %, 11 %, 40 %, 61 % and 67 % for first, second, third, fourth and fifth or more repeat caesarean deliveries, respectively [24].

The incidence of emergency peripartum hysterectomy is rising worldwide in view of the rising caesarean section rate and the concomitant rise in placenta praevia and placenta praevia accreta and multiple births [25].

5. Indications

Besides the predominant reported indications for emergency peripartum hysterectomy that include uterine atony, placenta praevia, placenta praevia accreta and uterine rupture, other reported risk factors include precipitate labour, induction, prolonged labour, dystocia, cephalopelvic disproportion, augmentation, foetal macrosomia, multiple pregnancy, retained products of conception, previous endometrial curettage, coagulopathy, thrombocytopenia, maternal obesity, advanced maternal age, previous primary postpartum haemorrhage, gestational diabetes and abruptio placentae, particularly the concealed variety that is associated with Couvelaire uterus. All were identified as independent risk factors for uterine atony [11-23].

Elective peripartum hysterectomy may be performed in patients with an antepartum diagnosis of placenta accreta or stage IA2 and IB1 cervical carcinoma [2]. Severe postpartum infection unresponsive to medical therapy and placental site vessel subinvolution are other potential indications for the procedure [26,27].

5.1. Postpartum haemorrhage

Severe post partum haemorrhage remains a significant cause of maternal morbidity and mortality in both developed and developing countries [28,29]. The rate of postpartum haemorrhage requiring blood transfusion was reported to occur in 1.7% deliveries [30]. Maternal complications of postpartum haemorrhage include hypovolaemic shock, disseminated intravascular coagulopathy (DIC), renal failure, hepatic failure and acute respiratory distress syndrome (ARDS) [31,32]. The most severe complication of haemorrhage is maternal death.

Haemorrhage, in general, is classified into four categories [33] (Table 1). Postpartum haemorrhage is measured by the loss of greater than 500 ml of blood following vaginal birth or 1000 ml of blood following caesarean section [34]. Postpartum haemorrhage can be minor (500–1000 ml) or major (more than 1000 ml). Major postpartum haemorrhage could be divided to moderate (1000–2000 ml) or severe (more than 2000 ml). A blood loss of more than 2000 ml is regarded as 'life threatening'.

Category	I	II	III	IV
Blood loss (ml)	<750	750–1500	1500–2000	>2000
Blood loss (%)	<15 %	15–30 %	30–40 %	>40 %
Pulse rate/min	<100	>100	>120	>140
Blood pressure	Normal	Hypo	Hypo	Hypo
Respiratory rate/min	14–20	20–30	30–40	>35
Urine output (ml/hour)	>30	20–30	5–15	<5
Signs and symptoms	None	Fatigue, pallor	Confusion	Life threatening
Action: stop loss	Observe	IV fluid	Blood transfusion	Blood transfusion

Table 1. Classification of haemorrhage

Haemorrhagic shock is a life-threatening condition that results when more than 20 % of the body's blood is lost. Symptoms include anxiety, blue lips and fingernails, low or no urine output, profuse sweating, tachypnoea, dizziness, confusion, chest pain, loss of consciousness, hypotension, tachycardia and weak pulse [35].

A Cochrane review addressed the use of uterotonics in the third stage of labour. It indicated that, for women delivering vaginally, oxytocin 5 IU by intramuscular injection is the regimen of choice for routine prophylaxis against postpartum haemorrhage. In the context of caesarean delivery, oxytocin 5 IU by intravenous injection is the recommended routine for prophylaxis against postpartum haemorrhage; the drug should be given slowly to avoid the risk of profound hypotension [36].

Drug	Route	Dose	Frequency
Oxytocin	IV	10–40 U in 1 L N saline	Continuous
Oxytocin	IM	10 U	
Ergometrine*	IM	0.5 mg	Every 2–4 h
PGF2α**	IM or intra-myometrially	0.25 mg	Every 15–90 min. Max. 8
PGE2	Vaginal or rectal	20 mg	Every 2 h
PGE1	Rectal	1 mg	

* Contraindicated in women with hypertension

** Contraindicated in women with asthma

Table 2. Pharmacological management of postpartum haemorrhage

To arrest postpartum haemorrhage, algorithms have been proposed to aid its systematic management. Procedures for immediate management of postpartum haemorrhage include the use of pharmacological uterotonic drugs (Table 2), uterine massage or bimanual uterine compression on an empty bladder, the initiation of blood and blood components therapy (Table 3), repair of genital tract lacerations, evacuation of retained products of conception, the implementation of uterine or internal iliac arteries or anterior division of internal iliac arteries embolisation (Figure 1), uterine tamponade techniques (Table 4) (Figure 2), uterine compression sutures (Figure 3), systematic pelvic devascularisation (Figure 4), internal iliac artery ligation (Figure 5) and recombinant-activated factor VII for category III and IV postpartum haemorrhage [37-44] . Consideration should be given to the possibility that placenta praevia percreta may extend into the bladder and other pelvic organs. Clinicians need to be aware of the appropriateness and the timing of instituting interventions.

Product	Volume	Contents	Effect [per unit]
Packed red cells	240 ml	RBC, WBC, plasma	Increase PCV 3 % points, Hb 1 g/dl
Platelets	50 ml	Platelets, RBC, WBC, plasma	Increase platelet 5,000–10,000/μl
Fresh frozen plasma	250 ml	Fibrinogen, antithrombin III, V, VIII	Increase fibrinogen by 10 mg/dl
Cryoprecipitate	40 ml	Fibrinogen, VIII, XIII, VWF	Increase fibrinogen by 10 mg/dl

Table 3. Blood component therapy

Modality	Method
Packing	4-inch gauze in 5 ml of sterile saline
Foley catheter	Insert one or more bulbs, instil 60–80 ml of saline
Sengstaken–Blakemore tube	
Tamponade balloon	Instil 300–500 ml of saline

Table 4. Uterine tamponade techniques for postpartum haemorrhage

Postpartum haemorrhage is a leading indication for emergency peripartum hysterectomy. Peripartum hysterectomy is generally performed in the setting of category IV life-threatening haemorrhage during or after abdominal and vaginal deliveries that cannot be controlled by the above medical and conservative surgical measures.

5.2. Uterine rupture

Uterine rupture is associated with maternal and perinatal mortality and morbidity worldwide, particularly in developing countries. The most common cause of uterine rupture is tear of a previous caesarean section scar after a trial of labour in a patient with a previous caesarean section. Rupture of an unscarred uterus is rare. It may occur in obstructed, multiparous labour and in response to inappropriate use of oxytocic agents. Its incidence decreases with improvement in obstetric practice [45].

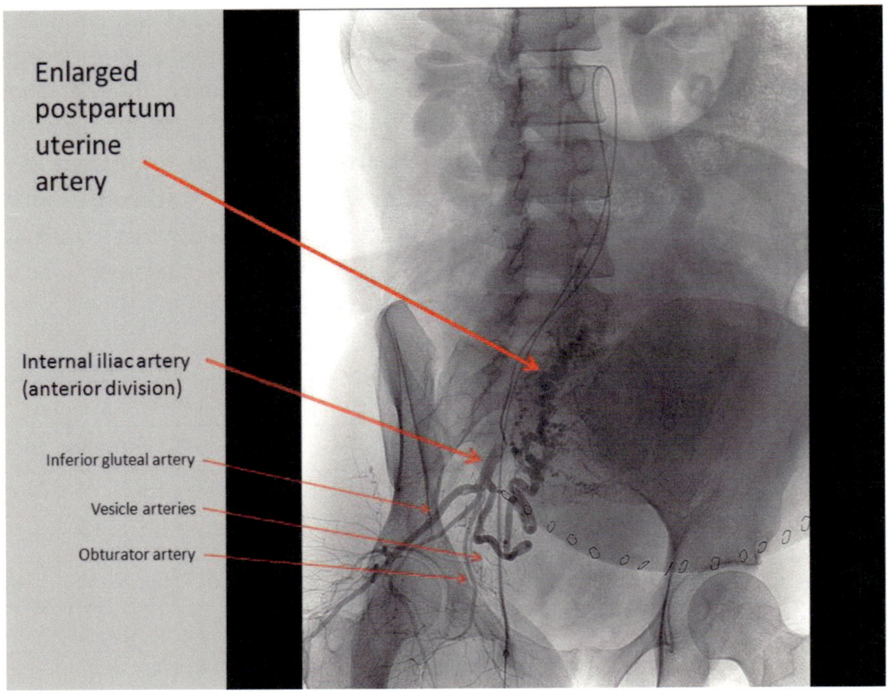

Figure 1. Internal iliac artery, anterior division angiogram. An enlarged uterine artery is present post-caesarean section. Courtesy of The Pump and the Tubes. A journal of all things vascular

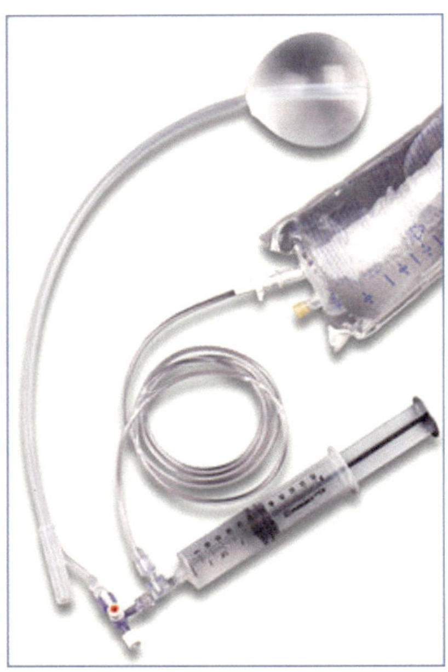

Figure 2. Uterine tamponade. Courtesy of Bt-Cath® With Easyfill™ Inflation System. Utah Medical Products, Inc.

http://dx.doi.org/10.5772/60942

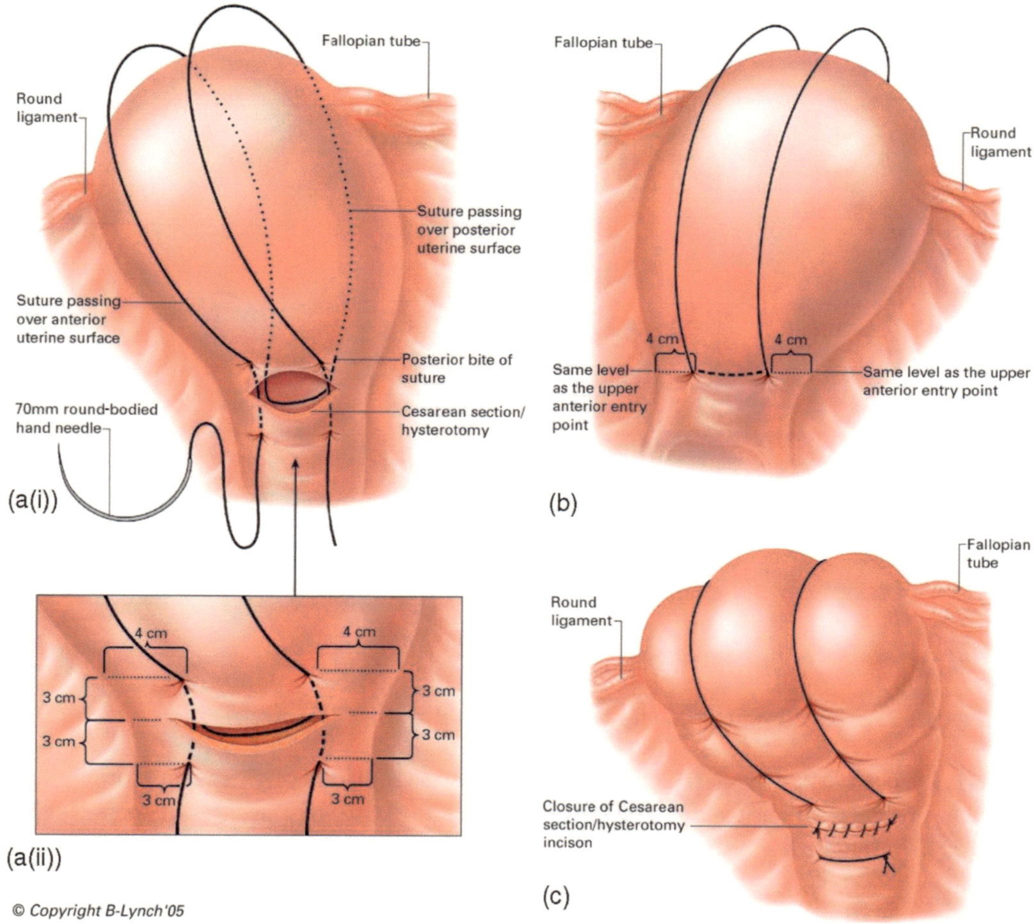

Figure 3. Uterine compression sutures. Courtesy of B-Lynch

Traumatic rupture can occur with internal version, classical application of the anterior blade of Kielland's forceps, manual removal of the placenta, manual exploration of the uterus and during curettage for secondary postpartum haemorrhage. Other causes of traumatic ruptures of the uterus are relatively rare and tend to occur at the fundus and usually result only from the most violent accidents [46].

5.3. Extension of the lower uterine segment incision

Caesarean hysterectomy may be necessary in cases of lateral extension of the lower uterine segment incision, when the caesarean section is performed with the foetal head deeply impacted in the pelvis in the second stage of labour. The tear may extend to branches of the uterine arteries. Haemostasis may be challenging; injuries to the ureters are possible. Broad ligament haematoma is not uncommon.

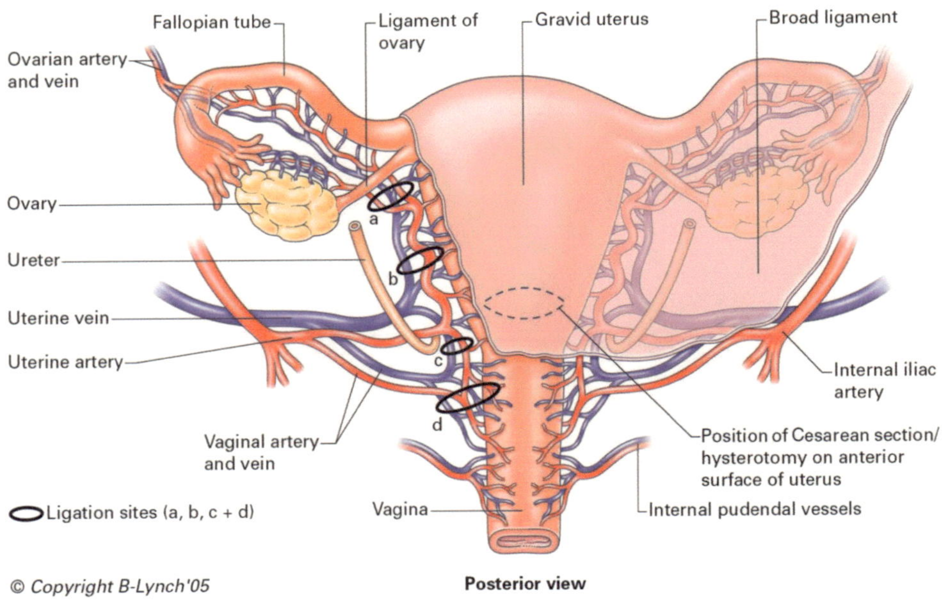

Figure 4. Stepwise devascularisation. Courtesy of B-Lynch

5.4. Uterine sepsis and placental site vessel subinvolution

Emergency peripartum hysterectomy may be necessary in cases of extensive uterine sepsis where antibiotic treatment is not effective and in the rare cases of placental site vessel subinvolution [27], in which uterine bleeding is protracted.

5.5. Abnormal placentation

The problems of uterine atony and uterine rupture have been greatly reduced through the use of potent uterotonic agents and the utilisation of modern obstetric care [47]. With the rising caesarean section rate and the rising incidence of placenta praevia and accreta and the more severe forms of increta and percreta, associated with previous caesarean sections, recent studies have indicated a change in the trend towards abnormal placentation (Figure 6) as the most common indication for emergency and planned peripartum hysterectomy [48-50]. In the absence of risk factors, early diagnosis of placental abnormalities is difficult. Unfortunately, the diagnosis is frequently established only after unsuccessful removal of the placenta at delivery.

5.5.1. Ultrasonography in the diagnosis of abnormal placentation

For the antenatal diagnosis of placenta accreta, transvaginal and transabdominal ultrasonography are complementary diagnostic techniques. Transvaginal ultrasound is safe for patients with placenta praevia. Normal placentation is characterised by a hypoechoic boundary between the placenta and the bladder. Features suggestive of placenta accreta include thinning

http://dx.doi.org/10.5772/60942

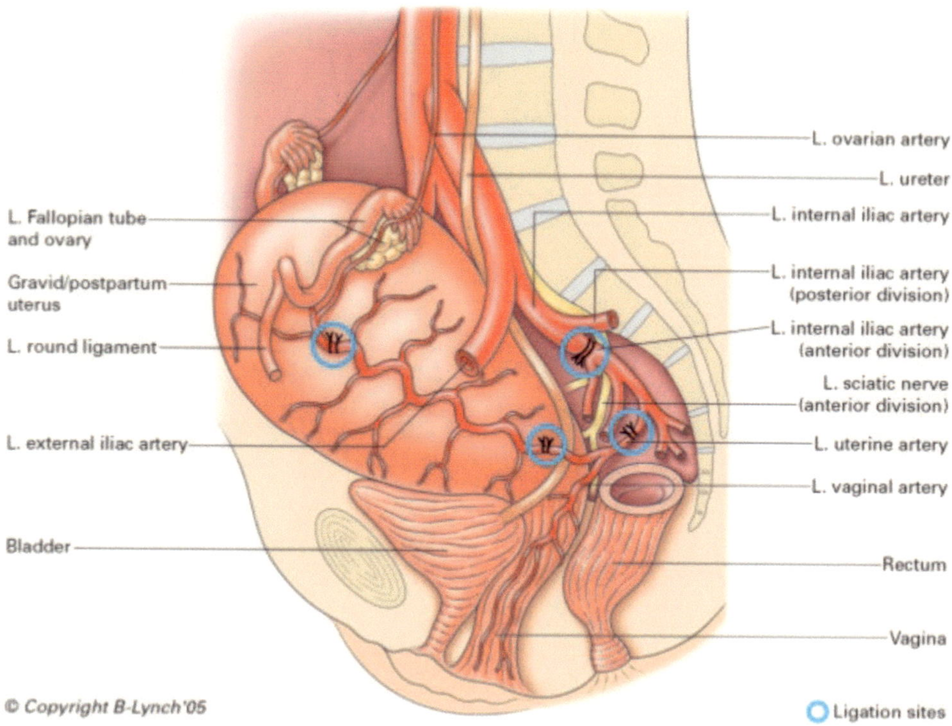

Figure 5. Systematic pelvic devascularisation and internal iliac artery ligation. Courtesy of B-Lynch

of the myometrium overlying the placenta (Figure 7), protrusion of the placenta into the bladder and irregularly shaped placental lacunae. The presence of lacunae 'moth-eaten or Swiss cheese appearance' within the placenta is predictive of placenta accreta (Figure 8). The use of colour Doppler, power Doppler or three-dimensional imaging may improve the diagnostic sensitivity (Figure 9), compared with that achieved by grayscale ultrasonography alone [51].

Overall, one study demonstrated that grayscale ultrasonography may be sufficient to diagnose placenta accreta, with a sensitivity of 91.4 % (95 % CI, 77.6–97.0 %), specificity of 95.9 % (95 % CI, 92.2–97.9 %), a positive predictive value of 80.0 % (95 % CI, 65.2–89.5 %) and a negative predictive value of 98.4 % (95 % CI, 95.5–99.5 %) [52]. Another study concluded that ultrasound for the prediction of placenta accreta may not be as accurate as previously described, with reported sensitivity, specificity, positive predictive value, negative predictive value and accuracy of 53.5 %, 88.0 %, 82.1 %, 64.8 % and 64.8 %, respectively [53].

5.5.2. Magnetic resonance imaging in the diagnosis of abnormal placentation

Magnetic resonance imaging (MRI) is considered to add little to the diagnostic accuracy of ultrasonography. However, when there are ambiguous ultrasound findings or a suspicion

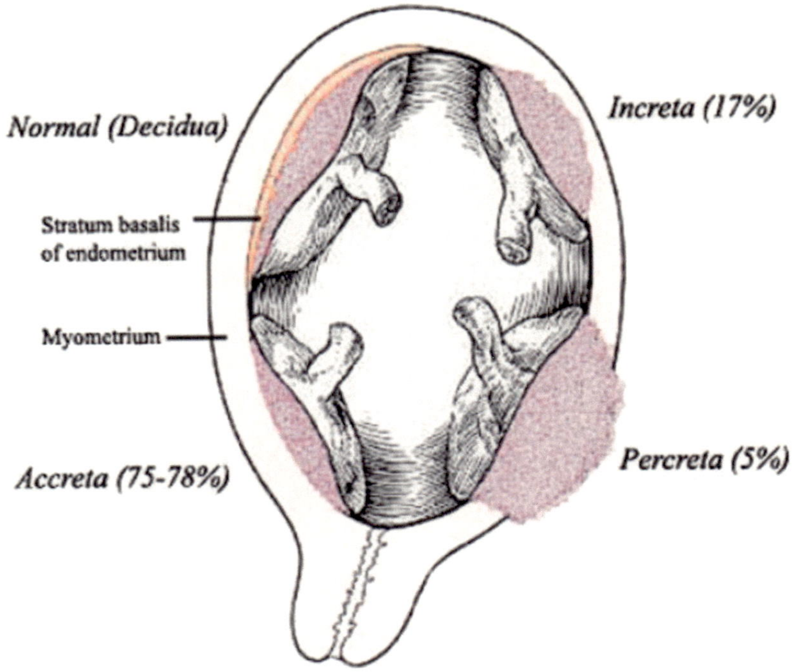

Figure 6. Diagram illustrating placenta accreta, increta and percreta. Courtesy of Callen P

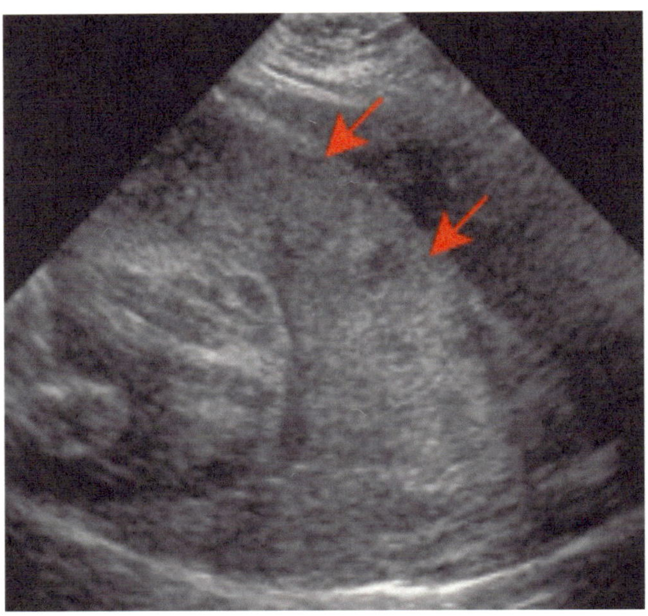

Figure 7. Sonogram demonstrating absence (arrows) of the intervening myometrium between the placenta and uterine serosa. Courtesy of Callen P

http://dx.doi.org/10.5772/60942

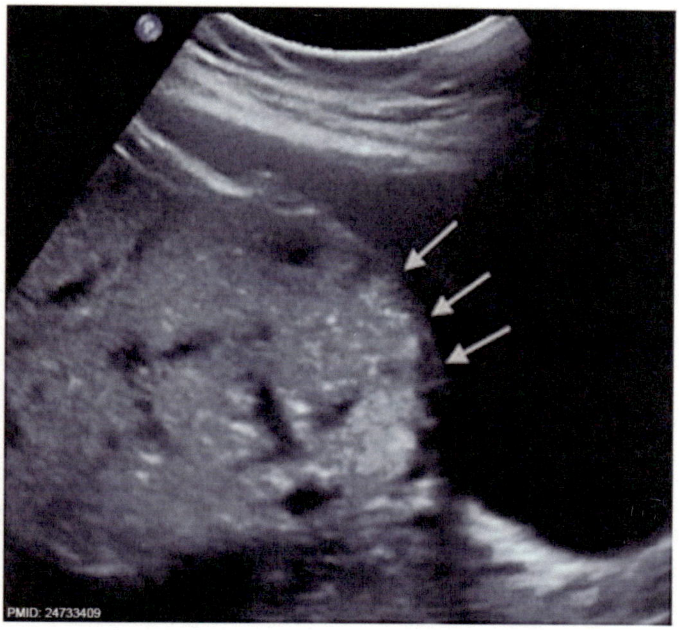

Figure 8. Sonogram demonstrating numerous vascular lacunae (arrows) within the placenta in a patient with placenta accreta Ultrasound of placenta and bladder wall interface indicating placenta accreta. Courtesy of Riteau et al.

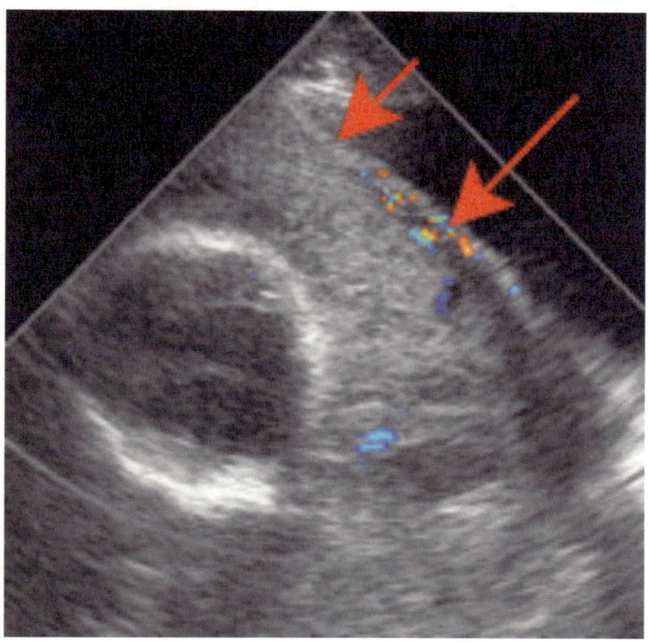

Figure 9. Colour Doppler image demonstrating absence of intervening myometrium (short arrow) and abnormal bladder–uterine wall vascularisation (long arrow). Courtesy of Callen P

of a posterior placenta accreta, with or without placenta praevia, ultrasonography may be insufficient. In general, MRI may better outline the anatomy and degree of invasion (Figure 10) [54].

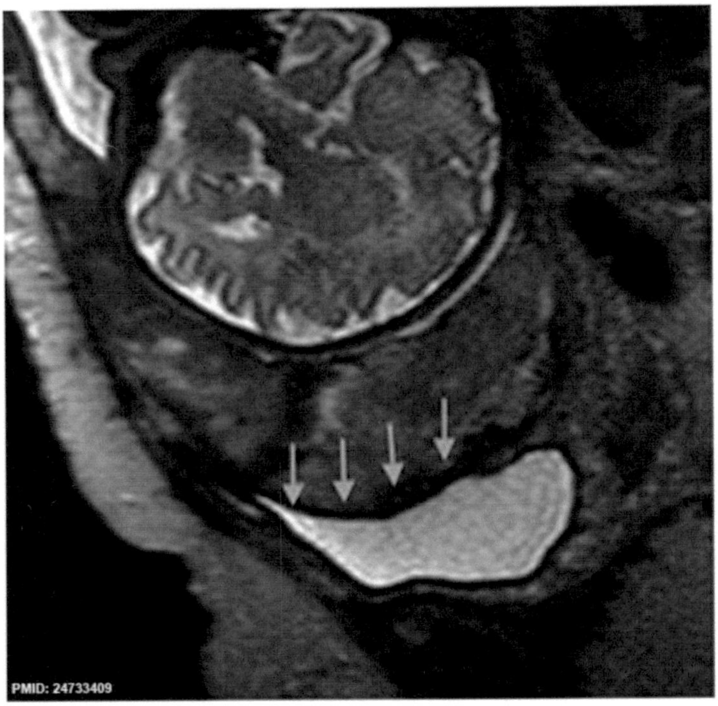

Figure 10. Sagittal magnetic resonance images indicated a bulge at the bladder wall indicating a major anterior placenta praevia accreta with bladder wall involvement. Courtesy of unsw.edu.au

Controversy surrounds the use of gadolinium-based contrast enhancement even though it adds to the specificity of the placenta accreta diagnosis by MRI. The use of gadolinium contrast enables MRI to more clearly delineate the outer placental surface relative to the myometrium. However, it is recommended that intravenous gadolinium should be used only if absolutely essential [55].

6. Prophylactic arterial occlusion

Recently, prophylactic arterial occlusion has been described as a strategy to reduce bleeding during planned hysterectomy (Figure 11). The efficacy and safety of this procedure is unknown. One small-scale study suggested that the successful use of a staged embolisation hysterectomy procedure for placenta accreta is associated with decreased maternal morbidity [56]. Another study using prophylactic intravascular balloon catheters did not benefit women

http://dx.doi.org/10.5772/60942

with placenta accreta undergoing caesarean hysterectomy [57]. The use of these procedures should not delay recourse to surgery.

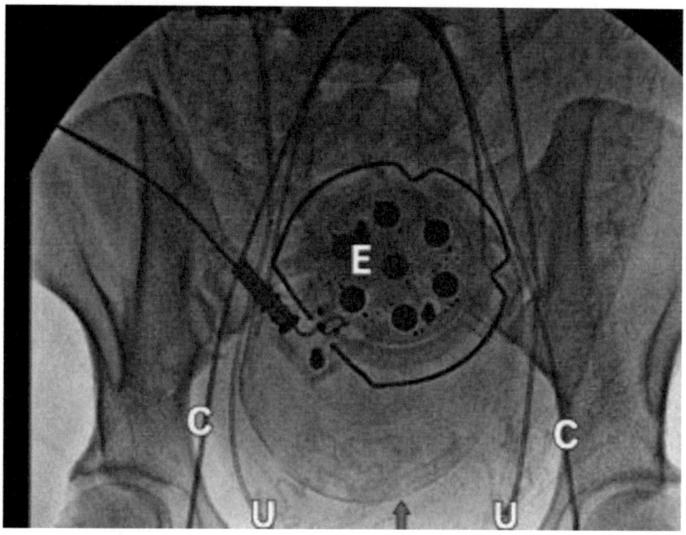

Figure 11. Placing arterial catheters (C) and ureteral catheters (U) preoperatively; E is the external foetal monitor. Courtesy of Ochsner 201

7. Preparation

Surgical planning is necessary. Once the decision is made to embark on surgical haemostasis, the most appropriate choice of procedure will depend on available resources and the expertise of available staff. Obstetricians should be prepared for the potential need to perform emergent peripartum hysterectomy. There is a high chance that a patient with uterine rupture, placenta accreta, increta or percreta will undergo hysterectomy [58]. At least 4 U of blood and blood products must be made available in suspected cases of accreta.

The acute loss of blood and the unplanned nature of surgery render the conditions for postpartum haemorrhage less than ideal to perform the procedure. Peripartum hysterectomy is associated with increased rates of both intraoperative and postoperative complications. Compared with nonobstetric hysterectomy, peripartum hysterectomy is associated with higher rates of morbidity and mortality. The mortality of peripartum hysterectomy is more than 25 times that of hysterectomy performed outside of pregnancy, with the higher rates in regions with limited medical and hospital resources [15]. Therefore, peripartum hysterectomy is considered a major dramatic life-saving surgical venture and represents the most challenging complication that an obstetrician will face.

Adequate resuscitation and prompt decision-making for hysterectomy would contribute to decreasing maternal morbidity and mortality, as timing is critical to an optimal outcome. It has been established that there is a relationship between the duration of time that passes prior to deciding to perform an emergency hysterectomy and the likelihood of coagulopathy, severe hypovolaemia, hypothermia and acidosis. Early recourse to hysterectomy is recommended, especially where bleeding is associated with placenta accreta or uterine rupture [59].

For peripartum hysterectomy, an experienced senior obstetrician with an experience in obstetric hysterectomy should be present at surgery. Of concern however is the limited experience of performing emergency hysterectomy among some obstetricians. Emergency peripartum hysterectomy being performed by an experienced surgeon is reported to significantly reduce maternal morbidity in general, operating time, number of units of blood transfusion and hospital stay in particular [60,61].

8. Other strategies for the management of abnormal placentation

Although hysterectomy has traditionally been advised for the management of placenta accreta, it is associated with considerable maternal morbidity and mortality. Therefore, new strategies have been attempted to manage this condition conservatively, so that fertility can be preserved and some of the complications of peripartum hysterectomy averted. Such strategies include leaving the placenta in situ, combined with uterine artery embolisation or uterine compression sutures, and the use of methotrexate to inhibit trophoblast growth. However, these conservative approaches may be limited by the high risk of bleeding, infection and poor placental absorption [62-64].

9. Transfusion-related acute lung injury as a major complication

Transfusion-related acute lung injury (TRALI) is a rare but potentially fatal complication of blood product transfusion, manifesting as acute respiratory distress syndrome (ARDS). It is characterised by acute respiratory distress following transfusion. All plasma-containing blood products have been implicated including rare reports of IVIG and cryoprecipitate. The symptoms typically develop during or within 6 h of a transfusion [32].

Transfusion-related acute lung injury patients present with the rapid onset of dyspnoea and tachypnoea. There may be associated fever, cyanosis and hypotension. Chest x-rays show bilateral patchy infiltrates, which may progress to the complete 'white out' oedema of acute respiratory distress syndrome.

It is hypothesised that transfusion-related acute lung injury may be precipitated by the infusion of donor antibodies directed against recipient leucocytes. The infusion of donor anti-HLA or anti-HNA antibodies is thought to directly cause complement activation, release of cytotoxic agents, endothelial damage and capillary leak. The majority of patients require ventilatory support [32].

Patients at high risk of caesarean hysterectomy should be scheduled for delivery at a time when appropriate ancillary staff with high-risk anaesthetists, interventional radiologists, urologists and resources is readily available. It is preferable to avoid emergency deliveries after the onset of labour, as the ancillary staff may not be available at a very short notice. Transfer of care to a tertiary care centre may be necessary if these resources are not locally available [65].

10. Counselling

Patients at risk for peripartum hysterectomy should be counselled about the likelihood of the procedure, what the procedure involves, complications, issues related to ovarian conservation and possible need for recovery in an intensive care unit. Forward planning for delivery highlights the importance of antenatal checks and screening to minimise blood loss, morbidity and mortality. After the initial postoperative recovery, women should receive a comprehensive outline of events from experienced obstetricians [66].

The fertility-ending nature of emergency obstetric hysterectomy can be devastating as some women that receive an emergency peripartum hysterectomy are primigravid. After the initial postoperative recovery, those women should be comprehensively counselled.

11. Types of hysterectomy and anaesthesia

Peripartum hysterectomy may be either subtotal or total. It has been recommended that the decision on the type of hysterectomy should be individualised. Subtotal hysterectomy may be preferable because it may be technically easier with shorter operating time, less blood loss, less urological injury and low morbidity, added to the fact that the cervix may be difficult to identify, especially if the patient has laboured and whose cervix is fully effaced, dilated and soft. This is important in the setting of severe acute haemorrhage [67,68].

In cases of placenta praevia, where the entire placental bed has to be removed, and if the lower segment, cervix and paracolpos are involved in the haemorrhage, total hysterectomy will be necessary for haemostasis. Similar approach is adopted for cases of placenta praevia accreta that is invading the cervical stroma.

In the preoperative preparation for peripartum hysterectomy, in suspected cases of accreta, 4 U of both packed red blood cells and plasma have to be cross-matched. Cryoprecipitate and platelets should be available. General anaesthesia is considered to be more appropriate when there is continuing bleeding and the cardiovascular stability is compromised.

When the cardiovascular is stable and there is no evidence of coagulation failure, regional anaesthesia can be used. This may be particularly appropriate where a working epidural has been in place during labour. A vertical skin incision should be considered to provide better exposure.

The technique of peripartum hysterectomy is similar in principle to that of abdominal hysterectomy in gynaecology, except for the anatomical and physiological changes in pregnancy that render the uterine and ovarian vessels enlarged and distended and the pelvic tissues oedematous and friable.

12. Intraoperative and postoperative complications

In some cases of peripartum hysterectomy, traumatised tissues at the base of the pelvis may continue to bleed following surgery despite ligation of obvious bleeding pedicles. This bleeding is usually associated with disseminated intravascular coagulation (DIC). In such cases, the application of pelvic pressure packs may provide haemostasis until haematological stability is achieved. Vascular embolisation may be considered in the interim [69].

In general, emergency procedures are associated with a higher rate of postoperative complications than planned procedures. Furthermore, compared with nonobstetric hysterectomy, peripartum hysterectomy is accompanied by substantial morbidity and mortality. The principal complications are febrile episodes, haemorrhage, urinary tract injuries, coagulopathy, paralytic ileus or bowel obstruction, wound sepsis/dehiscence, vaginal cuff bleeding, pulmonary embolism and the need for re-exploration because of persistent bleeding.

13. Morbidity and mortality

In a population-based analysis to examine the morbidity and mortality of peripartum hysterectomy in comparison with nonobstetric hysterectomy, bladder and ureteral injuries were more common for peripartum hysterectomy, 9 % compared with 1 % and 0.7 % compared with 0.1 % respectively, ($P<.001$). Rates of reoperation (4 % compared with 0.5 %), postoperative haemorrhage (5 % compared with 2 %), wound complications (10 % compared with 3 %) and venous thromboembolism (1 % compared with 0.7 %) were all higher in women who underwent peripartum hysterectomy. In multivariable analysis, the odds ratio for death from peripartum compared to nonobstetric hysterectomy was 14.4 (95 % confidence interval 9.84–20.98) [38].

During peripartum hysterectomy, scarring from previous caesarean sections may obliterate the utero-vesical pouch and make the dissection of the bladder from the uterus injury prone. Furthermore, the ureters may be sectioned, clamped or stitched because of heavy bleeding that interferes with proper exposure. The reported incidence of urological injuries with peripartum hysterectomy is high [38]. Within the context of the emergency situation and the available resources, it is best to diagnose and deal with any bladder or ureteric injury at the time of the hysterectomy. Any tear in the bladder should be repaired with two layers of 3/0 polyglactin (Vicryl) or equivalent suture. After repair of any bladder injury, the bladder can be filled with methylene blue or sterile milk to ascertain that this has been accomplished successfully. Perioperative cystoscopy with ureteral stent placement may be considered.

http://dx.doi.org/10.5772/60942

14. Technique

In the intraoperative stage of peripartum hysterectomy, the application of tourniquet around the uterine cervix can be attempted to reduce blood loss. This is facilitated by the use of transillumination, where the avascular spaces in the broad ligament, roughly opposite the level of a transverse lower caesarean incision, are identified and a catheter passed through on each side to encircle the lower uterine segment just above the cervix. The catheter should be twisted and tightly clamped. This would compress the uterine arteries. In addition, the application of straight clamps adjacent to the uterus to include the round ligaments, the Fallopian tubes and the utero-ovarian ligaments will serve to control the collateral blood flow to the uterus from the ovarian arteries. These two manoeuvres should occlude the main collateral ovarian and uterine artery supply to the uterus.

It is recommended that all pedicles should be doubly ligated in all types of hysterectomy. In peripartum hysterectomy, the vascular pedicles are particularly thick and oedematous. At first, a transfixing suture is applied, followed by an all encompassing ligature. Check should be made to ensure that there is no haematoma formation at the base of the pedicle.

In cases of hysterectomy for placenta praevia accreta, increta and percreta, the foetus is delivered through a classical uterine incision, and the intact placenta is left in situ while the hysterectomy is completed (Figure 12).

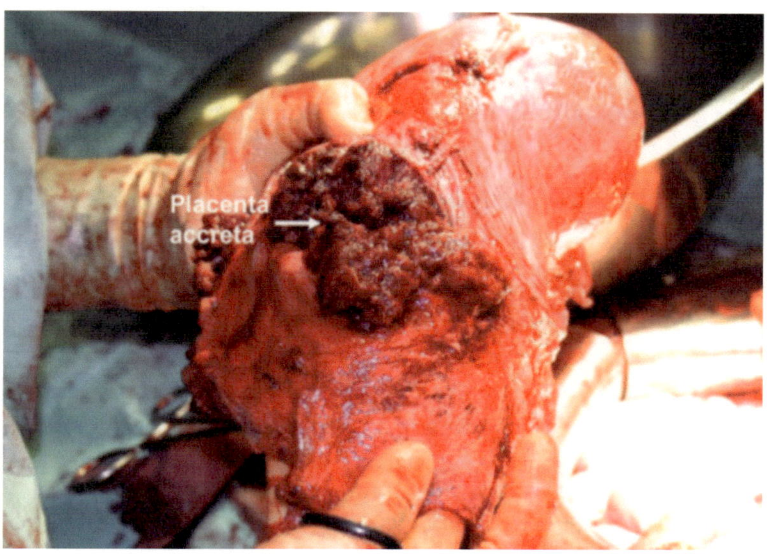

Figure 12. Hysterectomy specimen opened. Note placenta praevia percreta left in situ. © 2015 Callen P. Courtesy of Tikkanen, J Med Case Rep

At caesarean hysterectomy, a finger can be placed through the uterine incision and the cervical rim palpated. It is the safest to enter the vagina posteriorly, identify the rim of the cervix and then proceed anteriorly.

In general, No. 1 polyglactin (Vicryl) or equivalent is used throughout the peripartum hysterectomy procedures. Perioperative antibiotic prophylaxis should be continued for 24–48 h. Both mechanical and pharmacologic prophylaxis for deep venous thrombosis should be instituted. Thromboprophylaxis with heparin should be started as soon as one is satisfied that haemostasis is secure, at least 4 h postoperatively. The ovaries are almost always conserved. Peripartum hysterectomy is not a contraindication to breastfeeding. Women may use a breast pump temporarily until they are fit enough to breastfeed [70].

For an optimal management strategy for placenta accreta, it has been suggested that avoiding attempted placental removal at caesarean hysterectomy in women with suspected placenta accreta is associated with reduced maternal morbidity. Furthermore, some studies have recommended that patients with placenta accreta, increta or percreta who have no attempt to remove any of their placentae, with the aim of conserving their uterus, have reduced levels of haemorrhage and a reduced need for blood transfusion [62-64].

15. Recommendations

To provide a standardised approach to patients with postpartum haemorrhage, it is recommended that each labour unit should have a protocol for cases with estimated blood loss exceeding 1000 ml. Management involves four components that must be initiated simultaneously: communication, resuscitation, arresting the bleeding and monitoring and investigation, for optimal patient care. The following is a general guide for the management of major postpartum haemorrhage of more than 1000 ml and continuing to bleed OR clinical shock.

- Notify the senior obstetrician in charge, the department of anaesthesia, blood bank and laboratory.
- Establish two 14-gauge intravenous canula access; 20 ml blood sample should be taken for full blood count, coagulation screen, urea and electrolytes and cross match (4 U).
- For atony, administer oxytocin 10 IU by slow intravenous injection, followed by 40 IU in 500 ml of Hartmann's solution or normal saline at 125 ml/hour. If no intravenous access, give 10 IU intramuscularly. Oxytocin may be combined with other pharmacological agents; ergometrine 0.5 mg by slow intravenous or intramuscular injection (contraindicated in women with hypertension); carboprost 0.25 mg by intramuscular injection repeated at intervals of not less than 15 min to a maximum of eight doses (contraindicated in women with asthma); direct intramyometrial injection of carboprost 0.5 mg; misoprostol 1000 μg rectally (Table 2).
- Initiate uterine massage and/or manual uterine compression.
- Administer oxygen (10–15 l/min) by face mask or intubation, regardless of maternal oxygen concentration.
- Transfuse blood as soon as possible. If cross-matched blood is still unavailable, give uncross-matched group-specific blood or 'O RhD negative' blood. Four units of fresh frozen plasma

is given for every 6 U of red cells or prothrombin time/activated partial thromboplastin time more than 1.5 x normal (total 1 l). Platelet concentrates is administered if platelet count is less than 50 x 10^9/L and cryoprecipitate if fibrinogen is less than 1 g/L. The clinical picture should be the main determinant for the need for blood transfusion. Time should not be wasted waiting for laboratory results (Table 3).

- Until blood is available, infuse up to 3.5 L of warmed crystalloid Hartmann's solution (2 l) and/or colloid (1–2 l) as rapidly as required.
- Inspect the vagina and cervix for lacerations and repair them as necessary; evacuate any retained products of conception.
- If pharmacological measures fail to control the haemorrhage, initiate surgical haemostasis sooner rather than later. The following surgical interventions may be attempted, depending on clinical circumstances and available expertise:
  - Selective arterial embolisation
  - Uterine balloon tamponade (Table 4, Fig. 1)
  - Haemostatic brace suturing, such as B-Lynch or modified compression sutures
  - Bilateral ligation of uterine arteries
  - Bilateral ligation of internal iliac (hypogastric) arteries
  - Hysterectomy
- For the constant and close monitoring and support, unstable patients may need to be catered for in an intensive care unit.
- Common tests and their normal values include coagulation screen, electrolytes, liver function tests, acid-base and blood gases and kidney function tests (Table 5-9).

Test	Normal values
Platelet count (Plt)	140–450 x 10^3/μL
Mean platelet volume (MPV)	7.4–10.4 fL
Prothrombin time (PT)	1–15 s
International normalised ratio (INR)	0.9–1.2
Activated partial thromboplastin time (APTT)	18–45 s
Thrombin clotting time (TCT)	11–18 s
Fibrinogen	1.7–4.2 g/L
Antithrombin	0.15–0.39 mg/mL
Bleeding time	2–9 min
Viscosity	1.5–1.7 cP

Table 5. Coagulation-bleeding screen

Test	Normal value
Sodium (Na)	135–147 mEq
Potassium (K)	3.5–5 mEq
Bicarbonate (HCO_3)	24–30 mEq
Chloride (Cl)	100–106 mEq

Table 6. Electrolytes

Test	Normal value
ALT	5 to 56 U/L
AST	6 to 40 U/L
ALP	42 to 128 U/L
Total protein	35 to 84 g/L
Albumin	35 to 50 g/L
Globulins	25 to 35 g/L
Total bilirubin	0.1 to 1.0 mg/dL
Direct/conjugated bilirubin	0.0 to 0.4 mg/dL
GGT	9 to 48 U/L
LD	122 to 222 U/L
PT	9.5 to 13.8 s

Table 7. Liver function tests

Reports of balloon tamponade describe the intervention as the 'tamponade test'. Control of postpartum haemorrhage following inflation of the balloon indicates that laparotomy is not required. Continued postpartum haemorrhage following inflation of the balloon is an indication to proceed to laparotomy. This serves to affirm place of balloon tamponade as first-line procedure in the 'surgical' management of postpartum haemorrhage. The balloon should be left in place for 4–6 h, and, preferably, it should be removed during daytime hours. The balloon should be deflated and left in place for few minutes to ensure that bleeding does not reoccur [71,72].

The logistics for performing arterial occlusion or embolisation may not be readily available. This makes uterine balloon tamponade a more appropriate first-line treatment. Nevertheless, interventional radiology may be considered in cases of antenatal diagnosis of malplacentation, in the form of placenta praevia and placenta accreta, increta or percreta, where intra-arterial catheters, with the view of either occlusion or embolisation, can be placed prior to the performance of caesarean section. Follow-up studies of women who had undergone arterial embolisation or internal iliac artery ligation for control of postpartum haemorrhage suggest that these interventions do not impair subsequent menstruation, fertility and pregnancy outcomes [73,74].

Test	Arterial/venous	Normal values
pH	Arterial	7.35 to 7.45
	Venous	7.31 to 7.41
(H^+)	Arterial	36 to 44 nmol/L
		3.6 to 4.4 ng/dl
Base excess	Arterial and venous	-3 to +3 mEq/L
Oxygen partial pressure (pO_2)	Arterial	10 to 14 kPa
		75 to 105 mmHg
	Venous	4.0 to 5.3 kPa
		30 to 40 mmHg
Oxygen saturation (SpO_2)	Arterial	94 to 100 %
	Venous	Approximately 75 %
Carbon dioxide partial pressure (pCO_2)	Arterial	4.4 to 6.0 kPa
		33 to 45 mmHg
	Venous	5.5 to 6.8 kPa
		41 to 51 mmHg
Absolute content of CO_2	Arterial	23 to 30 mmol/L
		100 to 132 mg/dl
Bicarbonate (HCO_3)	Arterial and venous	18 to 23 mmol/L
		110 to 140 mg/dL
Standard bicarbonate (SBC)	Arterial and venous	21 to 28 mmol/L or mEq/L
		134 to 170 mg/dL

Table 8. Acid–base and blood gases

Test	Normal value
Blood urea nitrogen (BUN)	6 to 20 mg/dL
Creatinine	0.6 to 1.3 mg/dL
Urine creatinine (24-hour sample)	500 to 2000 mg/day. 11 to 26 mg/kg weight
Creatinine clearance	88 to 137 ml/min

Table 9. Kidney function tests

It recommended that these postpartum guidelines should be implemented at an estimated blood loss well below approx 2000 ml as the aim is to prevent haemorrhage escalating to the point where it is life threatening. In the face of relentless bleeding, up to 1 L of fresh frozen plasma and 10 U of cryoprecipitate (two packs) may be given while awaiting the results of coagulation studies. Factor VIIa therapy may be used as an adjuvant to standard pharmacological and surgical treatments, in a dose of 90 μg/kg, which may be repeated within 15–30 min in the absence of clinical response. Fibrinogen should be above 1 g/L and platelets greater than 20 x 109/L before Factor VIIa is given.

These recommendations are primarily for clinicians working in specialist-led obstetric departments; they are less appropriate for settings where resources are limited. It is recommended that the main therapeutic goals of management of massive blood loss are to maintain:

- Haemoglobin more than 8 g/dl
- Platelet count more than 75 x 10^9/L
- Prothrombin less than 1.5 x mean control
- Fibrinogen more than 1.0 g/L

Intraoperative cell salvage for autologous red cell transfusion is being investigated for use in obstetrics. The insertion of a central line will provide a means of accurate central venous pressure (CVP) monitoring and act as a route for rapid fluid replacement. In addition to central venous pressure line, a direct arterial pressure line should be used for cardiovascular monitoring in cases of major haemorrhage.

Increasing caesarean rates would lead to an increase in the number of peripartum hysterectomies for abnormal placentation. Because serious maternal morbidity and mortality increases progressively with increasing number of caesarean deliveries, the number of intended family size should be considered when counselling regarding elective primary caesarean delivery and elective repeat caesarean operation versus a trial of labour [73-76].

Peripartum hysterectomy is a challenging procedure. Its role in modern obstetrics is evolving. Improving management of postpartum haemorrhage should decrease peripartum hysterectomy for uterine atony. Peripartum hysterectomy merits a multidisciplinary approach.

Author details

Zouhair O. Amarin*

Address all correspondence to: zoamarin@hotmail.com

Faculty of Medicine, Mutah University, Karak, Jordan

References

[1] Smith J, Mousa HA. Peripartum hysterectomy for primary postpartum haemorrhage: incidence and maternal morbidity. J Obstet Gynecol. 2007;27:44-47.

[2] Ribeiro F, Correia L, Paula T, Santana I, Vieira Pinto L, Borrego J, Jorge AF. Cervical cancer in pregnancy: 3 cases, 3 different approaches. J Low Genit Tract Dis. 2013;17:66-70.

[3] Kwee A, Bots ML, Visser GH, Bruinse HW. Emergency peripartum hysterectomy: a prospective study in The Netherlands. Eur J Obstet Gynecol Reprod Biol. 2006;124:187-192.

[4] Elmir R, Schmied V, Wilkes L, Jackson D. Separation, failure and temporary relinquishment: women's experiences of early mothering in the context of emergency hysterectomy. J Clin Nurs. 2012;21:1119-1127.

[5] Lim WH, Pavlov T, Dennis AE. Analysis of emergency peripartum hysterectomy in Northern Tasmania. Aust J Rural Health. 2014;22:235-240.

[6] Umezurike CC, Adisa CA. Peripartum Hysterectomy. In: Al-Hendy A, Sabry M, editors. Hysterectomy. InTech Publishers; 2012. p. 83-102. DOI: 10.5772/34770, ch7

[7] Umezurike CC, Feyi-Waboso PA, Adisa CA. Peripartum hysterectomy in Aba Southeastern Nigeria. Aust Zeal J Obstet Gynecol. 2008;48:580-582.

[8] Whiteman MK, Kuklina E, Hillis SD, Jamieson DJ, Meikle SF, Posner SF, Marchbanks PA. Incidence and determinants of peripartum hysterectomy. Obstet Gynecol. 2006;108:1486-1492.

[9] Bassey G, Akani CI. Emergency peripartum hysterectomy in a low resource setting: a 5-year analysis. Niger J Med. 2014;23:170-175.

[10] Chawla J, Arora D, Paul M, Ajmani SN. Emergency Obstetric Hysterectomy: A Retrospective Study from a Teaching Hospital in North India over Eight Years. Oman Med J. 2015;30(3):181-186.

[11] Selo-Ojeme DO, Bhattacharjee P, Izuwa-Njoku NF, Kadir RA. Emergency peripartum hysterectomy in a tertiary London hospital. Arch Gynecol Obstet. 2005;271:154-159.

[12] Turner MJ. Peripartum hysterectomy: an evolving picture. Int J Gynecol Obstet. 2010;109:9-11.

[13] Allam IS, Gomaa IA, Fathi HM, Sukkar GF. Incidence of emergency peripartum hysterectomy in Ain-shams University Maternity Hospital, Egypt: a retrospective study. Arch Gynecol Obstet. 2014;290:891-896.

[14] Tikkanen M1, Paavonen J, Loukovaara M, Stefanovic V. Antenatal diagnosis of placenta accreta leads to reduced blood loss. Acta Obstet Gynecol Scand. 2011;90:1140-1146.

[15] Hall T, Wax JR, Lucas FL, Cartin A, Jones M, Pinette MG. Prenatal sonographic diagnosis of placenta accreta--impact on maternal and neonatal outcomes. J Clin Ultrasound. 2014;42:449-455.

[16] Baskett TF. Emergency obstetric hysterectomy. J Obstet Gynaecol. 2003;23:353–355.

[17] Bakshi S, Meyer BA. Indications for and outcomes of emergency peripartum hysterectomy. A five-year review. J Reprod Med. 2000;45:733-737.

[18] Glaze S, Ekwalanga P, Roberts G, Lange I, Birch C, Rosengarten A, Jarrell J, Ross S. Peripartum hysterectomy: 1999 to 2006. Obstet Gynecol. 2008;111:732-738.

[19] Habek D, Becareviç R. Emergency peripartum hysterectomy in a tertiary obstetric center: 8-year evaluation. Fetal Diagn Ther. 2007;22:139–142.

[20] Machado LS. Emergency peripartum hysterectomy: incidence, indications, risk factors and outcome. N Am J Med Sci. 2011;3:358–361.

[21] Begum M, Alsafi F, ElFarra J, Tamim HM, Le T. Emergency peripartum hysterectomy in a tertiary care hospital in Saudi Arabia. J Obstet Gynaecol India. 2014;64:321-327.

[22] Danisman N1, Kahyaoglu S, Celen S, Akselim B, Tuncer EG, Timur H, Kaymak O, Kahyaoglu I. The outcomes of surgical treatment modalities to decrease "near miss" maternal morbidity caused by peripartum haemorrhage. Eur Rev Med Pharmacol Sci. 2014;18:1092-1097.

[23] Bateman BT, Mhyre JM, Callaghan WM, Kuklina EV. Peripartum hysterectomy in the United States: nationwide 14 year experience. Am J Obstet Gynecol. 2012;206:63.e1-8.

[24] Silver RM, Landon MB, Rouse DJ, Leveno KJ, Spong CY, Thom EA, Moawad AH, Caritis SN, Harper M, Wapner RJ, Sorokin Y, Miodovnik M, Carpenter M, Peaceman AM, O'Sullivan MJ, Sibai B, Langer O, Thorp JM, Ramin SM, Mercer BM. Maternal morbidity associated with multiple repeat cesarean deliveries. Obstet Gynecol. 2006;107:1226-1232.

[25] Francois K, Ortiz J, Harris C, Foley MR, Elliott JP. Is peripartum hysterectomy more common in multiple gestations? Obstet Gynecol 2005;105:1369-372.

[26] Anderson BL. Puerperal group A streptococcal infection: beyond Semmelweis. Obstet Gynecol. 2014;123:874-882.

[27] Al-Mehaisen L, Al-Kuran O, Amarin ZO, Matalka I, Beitawi S, Muhtaseb A. Secondary postpartum haemorrhage following placental site vessel subinvolution: a case report. Arch Gynecol Obstet. 2008;278:585-587.

[28] Weeks A. The prevention and treatment of postpartum haemorrhage: what do we know, and where do we go to next? BJOG. 2015;122:202-210.

[29] Amarin Z, Khader Y, Okour A, Jaddou H, Al-Qutob R. National maternal mortality ratio for Jordan, 2007-2008. Int J Gynecol Obstet. 2010;111:152-156.

[30] Patterson JA, Roberts CL, Taylor LK, Ford JB. Reporting postpartum haemorrhage with transfusion: a comparison of NSW birth and hospital data. N S W Public Health Bull. 2014;24:153-158.

[31] Sakse A, Weber T, Nickelsen C, Secher NJ. Peripartum hysterectomy in Denmark 1995–2004. Acta Obstet Gynecol Scan. 2007;86:1472–1475.

[32] Teofili L, Bianchi M, Zanfini BA, Catarci S, Sicuranza R, Spartano S, Zini G, Draisci G. Acute lung injury complicating blood transfusion in post-partum haemorrhage: incidence and risk factors. Mediterr J Hematol Infect Dis. 2014;6:e2014069.

[33] Cababas JG, Manning JE, Cairns CB. Fluid and Blood Resuscitation. In: Tintinalli UE, Stapczynski JS, John Ma O, Cline DM, Cydulka RK, Meckler JD, editors. Tintinalli's Emergency Medicine: A Comprehensive Study Guide. 7th ed. McGraw-Hill: New York; 2004. p. 227, ch26.

[34] Creanga AA, Berg CJ, Syverson C, Seed K, Bruce FC, Callaghan WM. Pregnancy-related mortality in the United States, 2006-2010. Obstet Gynecol. 2015;125:5-12.

[35] Patil V, Shetmahajan M. Massive transfusion and massive transfusion protocol. Indian J Anaesth. 2014;58:590-595.

[36] British Medical Association; Royal Pharmaceutical Society of Great Britain. British National Formulary No. 57. London: BMJ Group and RPS Publishing [internet]. 2009 Available from http:// [www.bnf.org/bnf/bnf/57/4499.htm].

[37] Hoffman MS, Karlnoski RA, Mangar D, Whiteman VE, Zweibel BR, Lockhart JL, Camporesi EM. Morbidity associated with nonemergent hysterectomy for placenta accreta. Am J Obstet Gynecol. 2010;202:e1-e5.

[38] Wright JD, Devine P, Shah M, Gaddipati S, Lewin SN, Simpson LL, Bonanno C, Sun X, D'Alton ME, Herzog TJ. Morbidity and mortality of peripartum hysterectomy. Obstet Gynecol. 2010;115:1187-1193.

[39] Clausen C, Stensballe J, Albrechtsen CK, Hansen MA, Lönn L, Langhoff-Roos J. Balloon occlusion of the internal iliac arteries in the multidisciplinary management of placenta percreta. Acta Obstet Gynecol Scand. 2013;92:386-391.

[40] Agarwal N, Deinde O, Willmott F, Bojahr H, MacCallum P, Renfrew I, Beski S. A case series of interventional radiology in postpartum haemorrhage. J Obstet Gynaecol. 2011;31:499-502.

[41] Hatfield JL, Brumsted JR, Cooper BC. Conservative treatment of placenta accreta. J Minim Invasive Gynecol. 2006;13:510-513.

[42] Juneja SK, Tandon P, Mohan B, Kaushal S. A change in the management of intractable obstetrical haemorrhage over 15 years in a tertiary care center. Int J Appl Basic Med Res. 2014 Sep;4(Suppl 1):S17-9.

[43] Boynukalin FK, Boyar H, Gormus H, Aral AI, Boyar N. Bilateral hypogastric artery ligation in emergency setting for intractable postpartum hemorrhage: a secondary care center experience. Clin Exp Obstet Gynecol. 2013;40:85-88.

[44] Morel O, Perdriolle-Galet E, Mézan de Malartic C, Gauchotte E, Moncollin M, Patte C, Chabot-Lecoanet AC. Management of severe or persistent postpartum haemorrhage after vaginal delivery. J Gynecol Obstet Biol Reprod (Paris). 2014;43:1019-1029.

[45] Berhe Y, Wall LL. Uterine rupture in resource-poor countries. Obstet Gynecol Surv. 2014;69:695-707.

[46] Tweddale C. Trauma during pregnancy. Crit Care Nurs Q. 2006;29:53-67.

[47] Brown G, Allen L, Torkelson A. Direct patient interventions that can reduce maternal mortality in developing countries: a systematic review. Fam Med. 2013;45:550-557.

[48] Sakinci M, Kuru O, Tosun M, Karagoz A, Celik H, Bildircin FD, Malatyalioglu E. Clinical analysis of emergency peripartum hysterectomies in a tertiary center. Clin Exp Obstet Gynecol. 2014;41:654-658.

[49] Wani RV, Abu-Hudra NM, Al-Tahir SI. Emergency peripartum hysterectomy: a 13-year review at a tertiary center in Kuwait. J Obstet Gynaecol India. 2014;64:403-408.

[50] Bowman ZS, Eller AG, Bardsley TR, Greene T, Varner MW, Silver RM. Risk factors for placenta accreta: a large prospective cohort. Am J Perinatol. 2014;31:799-804.

[51] Cheung CS, Chan BC. The sonographic appearance and obstetric management of placenta accreta. Int J Womens Health. 2012;4:587–594.

[52] Chalubinski KM, Pils S, Klein K, Seemann R, Speiser P, Langer M, Ott J. Prenatal sonography can predict degree of placental invasion. Ultrasound Obstet Gynecol. 2013;42:518-524.

[53] Bowman ZS, Eller AG, Kennedy AM, Richards DS, Winter TC 3rd, Woodward PJ, Silver RM. Accuracy of ultrasound for the prediction of placenta accreta. Am J Obstet Gynecol. 2014;211:177.e1-7.

[54] Comstock CH, Bronsteen RA. The antenatal diagnosis of placenta accreta. BJOG. 2014;121:171-181.

[55] Garcia-Bournissen F, Shrim A, Koren G. Safety of gadolinium during pregnancy. Can Fam Physician. 2006;52:309-310.

[56] Angstmann T, Gard G, Harrington T, Ward E, Thomson A, Giles W. Surgical management of placenta accreta: a cohort series and suggested approach. Am J Obstet Gynecol. 2010;202:38.e1-9.

[57] Shrivastava V, Nageotte M, Major C, Haydon M, Wing D. Case-control comparison of cesarean hysterectomy with and without prophylactic placement of intravascular balloon catheters for placenta accreta. Am J Obstet Gynecol. 2007;197:402.e1-5.

[58] Eltabbakh GH, Watson JD. Postpartum hysterectomy. Int J Gynecol Obstet. 1995;50:257-262.

[59] Chestnut DH, Eden RD, Gall SA, Parker RT. Peripartum hysterectomy: a review of cesarean and postpartum hysterectomy. Obstet Gynecol. 1985;65:365-370.

[60] Fitzpatrick KE, Sellers S, Spark P, Kurinczuk JJ, Brocklehurst P, Knight M. The management and outcomes of placenta accreta, increta, and percreta in the UK: a population-based descriptive study. BJOG. 2014;121:62-70.

[61] Ibrahim M, Ziegler C, Klam SL, Wieczorek P, Abenhaim HA. Incidence, indications, and predictors of adverse outcomes of postpartum hysterectomies: 20-year experience in a tertiary care centre. J Obstet Gynaecol Can. 2014;36:14-20.

[62] Torrenga B, Huirne JA, Bolte AC, van Waesberghe JH, de Vries JI. Postpartum monitoring of retained placenta. Two cases of abnormally adherent placenta. Acta Obstet Gynecol Scand. 013;92:472-475.

[63] Eller AG, Porter TF, Soisson P, Silver RM. Optimal management strategies for placenta accreta. BJOG. 2009;116:648-654.

[64] Eller AG, Bennett MA, Sharshiner M, Masheter C, Soisson AP, Dodson M, Silver RM. Maternal morbidity in cases of placenta accreta managed by a multidisciplinary care team compared with standard obstetric care. Obstet Gynecol. 2011;117:331-337.

[65] Silver RM, Fox KA, Barton JR, Abuhamad AZ, Simhan H, Huls CK, Belfort MA, Wright JD. Center of excellence for placenta accreta. Am J Obstet Gynecol. 2014;20. pii: S0002-9378(14)02248-0.

[66] de la Cruz CZ, Coulter ML, O'Rourke K, Amina Alio P, Daley EM, Mahan CS. Women's experiences, emotional responses, and perceptions of care after emergency peripartum hysterectomy: a qualitative survey of women from 6 months to 3 years postpartum. Birth. 2013;40:256-263.

[67] Amarin Z. Subtotal Versus Total Abdominal Hysterectomy for Benign Gynecological Conditions. In: Al-Hendy A, Sabry M, editors. Hysterectomy. InTech Publishers; 2012. p. 23-29. DOI: 10.5772/34770, ch2.

[68] Yoong W, Massish N, Oluwu A. Obstetric hysterectomy: changing trends over 20 years in a multiethnic high risk population. Arch Gynecol Obstet. 2006;274:37-40.

[69] Izbizky G, Meller C, Grasso M, Velazco A, Peralta O, Otaño L, Garcia-Monaco R. Feasibility and safety of prophylactic uterine artery catheterization and embolization in the management of placenta accreta. J Vasc Interv Radiol. 2015;26:162-169.

[70] Olza-Fernández I, García-Murillo L, Palanca-Maresca I. Breastfeeding following emergency peripartum hysterectomy. Breastfeed Med. 2012;7:307-309.

[71] Condous GS, Arulkumaran S, Symonds I, Chapman R, Sinha A, Razvi K. The 'tamponade test' in the management of massive postpartum haemorrhage. Obstet Gynecol. 2003;101:767-772.

[72] Frenzel D, Condous GS, Papageorghiou AT, McWhinney NA. The use of the 'tamponade test' to stop massive obstetric haemorrhage in placenta accreta. BJOG. 2005;112:676-677.

[73] Tadesse W, Farah N, Hogan J, D'Arcy T, Kennelly M, Turner MJ. Peripartum hysterectomy in the first decade of the 21st century. J Obstet Gynaecol. 2011;31:320-321.

[74] Daskalakis G, Anastasakis E, Papantoniou N, Mesogitis S, Theodora M, Antsaklis A. Emergency obstetric hysterectomy. Acta Obstet Gynecol Scand. 2007;86:223-227.

[75] Nizard J, Barrinque L, Frydman R, Fernandez H. Fertility and pregnancy outcomes following hypogastric artery ligation for severe post-partum haemorrhage. Hum Reprod. 2003;18:844-848.

[76] Salomon LJ, deTayrac R, Castaigne-Meary V, Audibert F, Musset D, Ciorascu R, et al. Fertility and pregnancy outcome following pelvic arterial embolization for severe post-partum haemorrhage. A cohort study. Hum Reprod. 2003;18:849-852.